THE MODERN VIKING DIET

A Practical Guide to Reclaim Your Health in a Toxic World

DR. LAURA CAPINA

Foreword by
DAVID WOLFE

Copyright © 2025, Dr. Laura Capina
Synerchii
All rights reserved.

ISBN: 979-8218836375

Produced by Publish Pros | publishpros.com

This book is not intended to diagnose, treat, cure, or prevent any disease. The information provided is based on the author's professional experience, personal research, and traditional wellness practices. It is not a substitute for medical advice from a licensed healthcare provider.

Always consult with your physician or qualified health practitioner before beginning any dietary, detox, or lifestyle change, especially if you are pregnant, nursing, have a medical condition, or are taking medications.

The author and publisher disclaim any liability for adverse effects resulting from the use of the information contained in this book.

Statements in this book have not been evaluated by the Food and Drug Administration.

DEDICATION

To my ancestors—
Who sang through oppression, danced through sorrow, and passed down wisdom in whispers and rituals.
Your resilience lives in my bones.
Your courage lights the path I now walk.

To my son, Matei—
May you grow strong in body, clear in mind, and rooted in truth.
May you remember who you are, and who you come from.
This is my prayer for you: to live as fully, freely, and vibrantly as the wild Viking heart that beats in your blood.

To the future generations—
May this book be a torch passed forward,
A guide to remember what was once forgotten,
And a reminder that true health is not found in fads or fear,
But in the deep, ancient rhythms of nature, nourishment, and purpose.

TABLE OF CONTENTS

Foreword · vii
Preface · xi
Introduction · xv

The Viking Lifestyle · 1
The Viking Diet—Fuel of Warriors · 5
Core Principles · 15
    Eat Real, Whole, Wild Food · 15
    Nourish Your Cells with Omega3s · · · · · · · · · · · · · · · · · · 17
    Master Blood Sugar · 20
    Cycle Fasting and Feasting · 27
    Focus on Bitter, Fermented, and Wild Foods · · · · · · · · · 41
    Let Food Be Your Medicine · 49
    Live with Rhythm · 61
    Live with Purpose, Intention, and Ancestral Meaning · · · · · · · 74
    The Non-negotiables · 80
Detox like a Viking · 85
    Colon and Intestinal Cleanse · 86
    Liver and Gallbladder Flush · 91
    Kidney and Bladder Cleanse · 96
    Heavy Metal Detox · 100

- Parasite Cleanse · 104
- Spike Protein and Synthetic Toxin Cleanse · · · · · · · · · · · · · 110
- Lymph and Skin Detox · 115
- Mold Toxicity · 118
- Glyphosate · 121

Viking Superfoods, Herbs, and Modern Power Nutrients · · · · · · 129
Daily Rituals of the Modern Viking · 139
Recapturing Calm · 145
The Longevity Code · 151
Viking Diet Recipes · 169
Plant-Based Power—the Viking Diet for Vegans · · · · · · · · · · · · · 205
What Should I Eat? Personalized Nutrition · · · · · · · · · · · · · · · · 225
The Path Forward · 235

FOREWORD

David "Avocado" Wolfe
Author, Orator, Organic Farmer, Adventurer

As you will discover within these pages, The Viking Diet was shaped by the raw elements of the Scandinavian and North Atlantic environment. The quasi-agrarian lifestyle, wild-food foraging, and seafaring expeditions of this amazing culture always gave them some source of vital nourishment. Their system was practical, sustainable, and deeply influenced by the availability of local resources, seasonal changes, and preservation techniques necessary for long winters and voyages.

The Vikings valued food as a fuel for survival and as a source of ancestral and spiritual strength, so much so, that they would risk boarding cows, sheep, chickens, cats, dogs, and even horses on their ships to recreate their food, home-building, and survival strategies abroad.

The Viking Diet consisted of a wide variety of plant, animal, mushroom, and fermented food sources. Their diet offered a balance of protein, fat, and carbohydrates to support a physically demanding lifestyle in climates as extreme as humans can survive in. Feasting was also a cultural cornerstone, symbolizing community, status, and celebration, where food was shared generously, often accompanied by mead (honey wine) or ale. The philosophy was a pragmatic one: Eat what the land and sea provide, preserve efficiently, and adapt to scarcity or abundance. They would often cycle between fasting and feasting.

The Vikings seized the day. They were a beautiful and adventurous people. To them, every day was the best day ever!

Personally, I have always felt an intense kinship with the Vikings: their lifestyle, beauty, history, pantheon of deities, spirit of adventure, and impact on the world. Their culture is vast and deeply fascinating to me. Leading to over thirty trips to Iceland and trips to Scandinavia at least a half a dozen times, I currently grow numerous Nordic plants and live in a Nordic environment part of each year. Nordic lifestyle concepts such as hot saunas, cold water plunging, wild berries for healing, the power of spring water, etc. have always been appealing and fit into my love of healing and healing strategies in general.

As an example, I have been so impacted by The Viking mariners and their super-vitamin C-rich berry, the sea buckthorn berry, I set about growing these on my farm in Northern Ontario, Canada. The Vikings never succumbed to scurvy—unlike many British sailors who followed in their wake. Why? Because The Vikings had a diet rich in sea buckthorn berries, whose vitamin C prevented scurvy. And they knew what was in those berries was important enough to take the plant to Iceland (as I have personally seen) and theoretically beyond to Greenland and North America.

Did you know The Vikings could sail up onto a beach in North America and begin smelting iron from iron-rich swamps by creating a bloomery—a portable, small-scale iron smelting furnace—made of clay, straw, and sand? They would take the iron-rich dirt from the swamp, cook it down with charcoal right on the beach, and produce enough iron slag to be poured into molds. They made axe heads, arrowheads, tools, swords, weapons, chain mail, horse fittings, ingots, and other items essential for their survival, trade, and warfare.

The bloomery's versatility allowed Vikings to produce iron goods tailored to their immediate needs. The quality and output depended on the smith's skill and available natural resources. Isn't that fascinating? I found it incredible that The Viking expeditions had this innate capability to source iron from the environment and make things out of iron quickly! I have never met anyone who has those skills today!

Upon contemplation of these interesting people, one is left wondering how the lessons of The Vikings may touch us today.

As you read this book, and as part of your continuing investigation into the Modern Viking Diet, please visit a local Nordic spa. And if you can get there, soak in a hot spring or two in Iceland; visit the fjords in Norway; forage wild mushrooms in Sweden; swim in a wild lake in Latvia.

In a world where attacks are coming from all sides—toxic food, contaminated water, noxious air, electromagnetic smog, sedentary lifestyles, etc.—it is smart to access the ferocity and also the flexibility of the Vikings to combat all of these and come out looking gorgeous and victorious. That is The Modern Viking Diet and wisdom of these pages in a nutshell.

The gifts of the Vikings and their culture are still around and now readily accessible in the pages of this book. Enjoy the knowledge, insights, and recipes you'll find here. Take what is ancient and make it brand new in your life. Nourish your vitality. It's time to take action in the direction of your dreams.

PREFACE

Your blood remembers what the world forgot. It's time to awaken the ancient strength within.

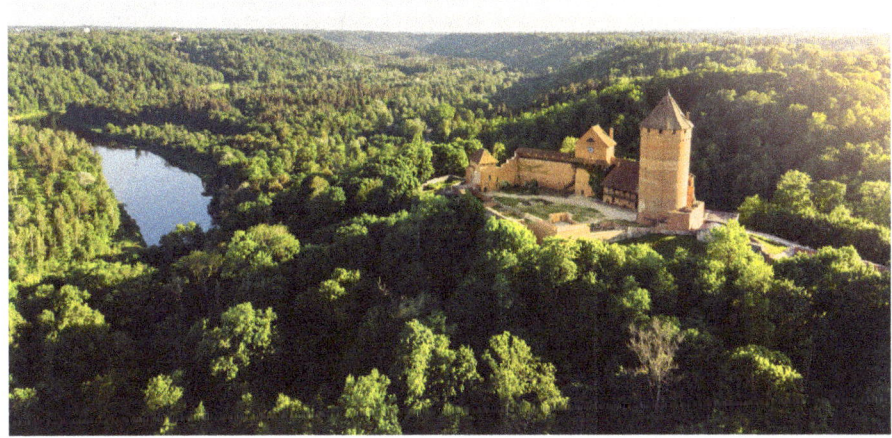

I was born and raised in Latvia, a small country in northeastern Europe on the Baltic Sea. With its beautiful forests and lakes, and deep traditions, my birthplace is more Scandinavian in spirit than many realize. However, I grew up under the cloud of Soviet occupation, in an era of scarcity and survival. We didn't have much, but we drew strength from our culture, community, and connection to nature.

We lived in Riga, the capital—a breathtaking city with cobblestone streets and old-world charm—but every summer I escaped to my aunt's rural home or my uncle's river house where life flowed with the rhythm of water and wildness. Those summers live in my bones. We swam, picked berries straight from the bushes, and cooked mushrooms we foraged ourselves. My uncles were master fishermen, and we feasted on fresh, smoked, stewed, and marinated fish. Everything we ate came from the earth or water around us, and nature was full of medicinal treasures—chaga mushrooms, nettle, meadowsweet, calendula, chamomile. We'd tap birch trees and drink their sap to rejuvenate our bodies. When we felt unwell, we reached first for herbs and teas. Pharmaceuticals were a last resort.

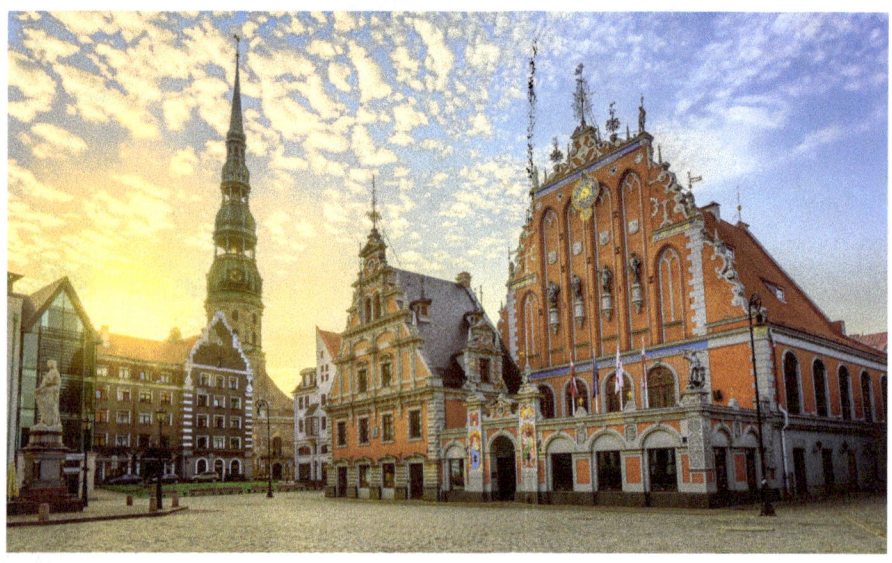

That was my normal. So imagine my shock when, in my early twenties, I moved to the United States and witnessed a very different world. People everywhere—young and old—were suffering from obesity, allergies, chronic illness, autism, anxiety, depression . . . I had never seen anything like it growing up. It sparked a fire in me: *Why? Why are people in the most developed country in the world so sick, tired, and disconnected?*

That question led me on a lifelong quest to understand health from every angle. I earned a master's and doctorate in Traditional Chinese Medicine and even went to China to study with traditional doctors to learn firsthand how ancient practices could heal what modern medicine often overlooks.

For nearly two decades now, I've treated thousands of patients with acupuncture, herbal medicine, nutritional guidance, and testing. And one thing has become crystal clear—the modern world has deviated dangerously far from nature and from God's design: Much of what we call food today is a chemical-laced imitation—void of real nourishment, yet disguised as sustenance. Our soil is depleted. Our air is polluted. Our minds are overstimulated, and our bodies are undernourished. That's why regular detox is no longer a luxury; it's a biological necessity in today's world. But detox alone isn't enough. What you eat every day either fuels disease or builds resilience. And yet, when it comes to nutrition, the confusion is everywhere. From vegan to carnivore, Mediterranean to keto, everyone claims to have the answer. So how do you know what's right for you?

I've studied nearly every major diet. I've researched their philosophies, studied their science, and observed their outcomes in real patients. What I discovered is that many of these diets have some truth—but most are too extreme, restrictive, or incomplete. That's what led me to create *The Modern Viking Diet*, a common-sense,

God-designed, science-backed lifestyle that reflects how the body is truly meant to function. It honors nature, ancestral wisdom, and modern research. It's not about extremes, it's about connecting back to the source—and it's the only path I've found that consistently restores strength, energy, and long-term health.

INTRODUCTION

*In a world that profits from your weakness,
reclaiming your strength is an act of rebellion.*

RECLAIMING STRENGTH IN A TOXIC WORLD

The Vikings drank clean water from streams, breathed crisp northern air, and ate real food. Every part of their lifestyle was cleansing, nourishing, and strengthening. Fast forward to today ... and we are living in a very different world.

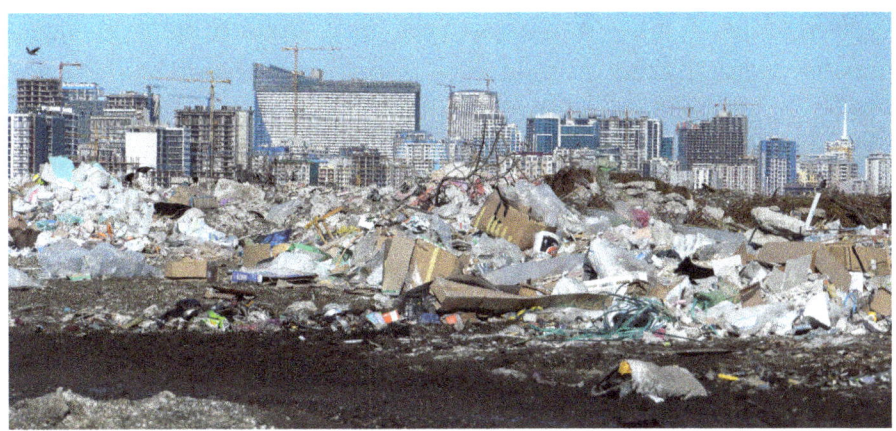

Our modern environment is a minefield of chemicals and heavy metals, electromagnetic pollution, endocrine disruptors, artificial light, and chronic stress. Modern diets rely heavily on processed foods—many of which are genetically modified, pesticide-laden, and nutritionally depleted. Our gut microbiomes are wrecked. And our bodies—biologically wired for the ancient world—are struggling to keep up. We've traded resilience for convenience, vitality for vanity, and instinct for programming.

And the consequences? They're everywhere. Obesity, autoimmune disease, infertility, brain fog, allergies, chronic fatigue, hormonal chaos, depression, anxiety, cancer. These are not random. They are symptoms of disconnection—from nature, from wisdom, from our ancestral roots. But you can get that power back.

To thrive in this toxic world, we need to bring the Viking spirit forward. We need to reclaim the strength of body that comes from real food and functional movement; the clarity of mind that comes from a clean gut, a nourished brain, and a connected soul; and the purity of purpose that comes from living in alignment with something greater than ourselves.

The Modern Viking Diet is not just a way of eating, it is a full system of living. It's a map back to yourself, a blueprint for navigating the chaos, based on nine core principles outlined in the Core Principles chapter.

To understand why this new Viking way is essential, you should know what modern Vikings are fighting:

- Toxins in our food, water, cosmetics, air, and even clothing
- Microplastics that have been detected in our blood, lungs, and even placentas
- Heavy metals like mercury, lead, and aluminum accumulating in our brains and bones

- Endocrine disruptors (from plastics and chemicals) wreaking havoc on our hormones
- Gut dysbiosis due to antibiotics, pesticides, processed foods, and sugar
- EMFs and blue light altering our circadian rhythms and damaging mitochondria
- Stress draining our adrenals and weakening immunity

The old "calories in, calories out" model simply doesn't cut it anymore. This is a war on vitality. But you're a Viking. You're built for this.

ANCIENT BLUEPRINT, MODERN ARMOR

This book will guide you to combine the resilient lifestyle of the ancient Norse, nutritional intelligence of the most effective diets in history, along with the discoveries and cutting-edge science of what actually has proven to be effective, and detox strategies of modern functional medicine and ancient herbalism.

We'll talk about how to eat, cleanse, train, think, and live—not just to survive in this modern world but to dominate it. Because the truth is, this toxic world isn't going to get easier. You just have to get stronger. And strength is built—not just in the gym—but in your kitchen, your bedroom, your mindset, your habits, your detox rituals, and your connection to nature and purpose.

You don't need to go back in time to be strong like a Viking. You need to go forward with ancient power in your hands and modern tools in your pack.

Let me show you how.

THE VIKING LIFESTYLE

Strength is not just in the muscle—but also in the mind, the gut, and the spirit.

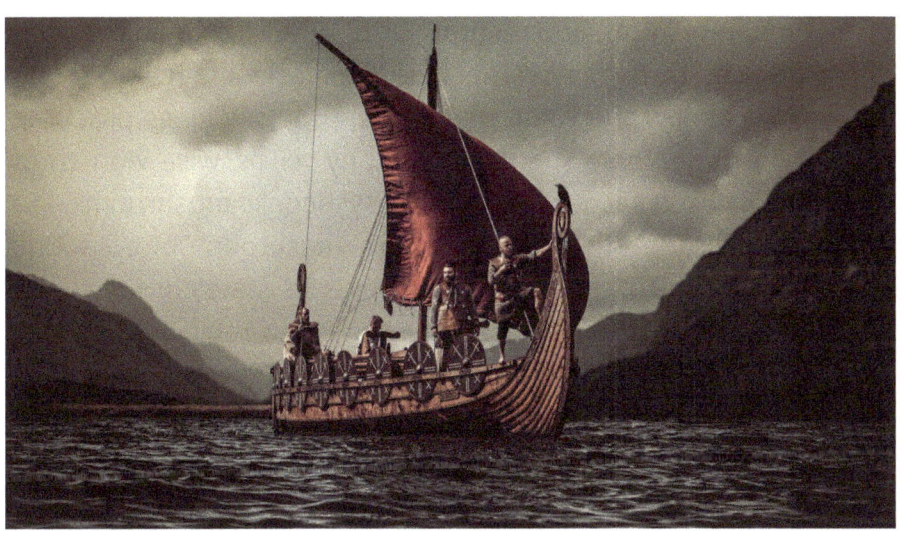

"Viking" brings to mind images of fierce warriors, longships slicing through icy waters, and brutal raids, but Vikings were much more than raiders and conquerors. They were healers, mystics, and masterful navigators of both land and spirit. They were deeply connected to nature and lived in rhythm with the seasons.

The Viking body was not chiseled in the gym—it was forged in the elements. They were lean, strong, fast, and functional. Their health and vitality didn't come from supplements or fitness trackers. It came from living hard, working with their hands, and eating real food. They didn't need motivation to move—they moved to survive.

They lived a detoxed lifestyle, eating what was local and seasonal—fresh-caught fish, grass-fed meats and wild game, root vegetables and greens, seaweed, berries, medicinal herbs and wild mushrooms—and drinking mead made from fermented honey.

They also fasted naturally, often going without food for long periods while traveling or working. They had to adapt. Their digestion, immune systems, and mental clarity were all shaped by cycles of feasting and fasting, movement and rest, cold and heat.

And they knew the value of spiritual rituals. Vikings practiced *seidr*—a form of Norse shamanism led by *völvas*, wise women or seers. *Völvas* used sacred plants and psychedelic mushrooms, like Amanita muscaria—the red-and-white mushroom often found beneath trees—to open gateways to altered states, visions, and deep ancestral wisdom. These experiences weren't recreational. They were rites of power and communion, used for divination, healing, and receiving guidance from their gods and ancestors. Fire, chanting, drumbeats, fasting, and isolation in nature were also used to open the veil between worlds.

Viking spirituality was deeply woven into every meal, every hunt, every storm and sunrise. They believed in fate (*Wyrd*), in the strength of their lineage, and in living a life worthy of their ancestors' honor. They lived in a way that kept them close to the earth, close to spirit, and close to their inner power.

That's what we've lost in the modern world—and what we're here to reclaim. *The Modern Viking Diet* is about more than food.

It's about stepping back into that legacy of balance, strength, and deep connection—to the body, the earth, and the wild self within. However, before we delve deeper into the Viking lifestyle—and the other core principles of the Viking diet—let's talk about food first!

THE VIKING DIET—FUEL OF WARRIORS

Every bite you take is a choice—toward healing or away from it.

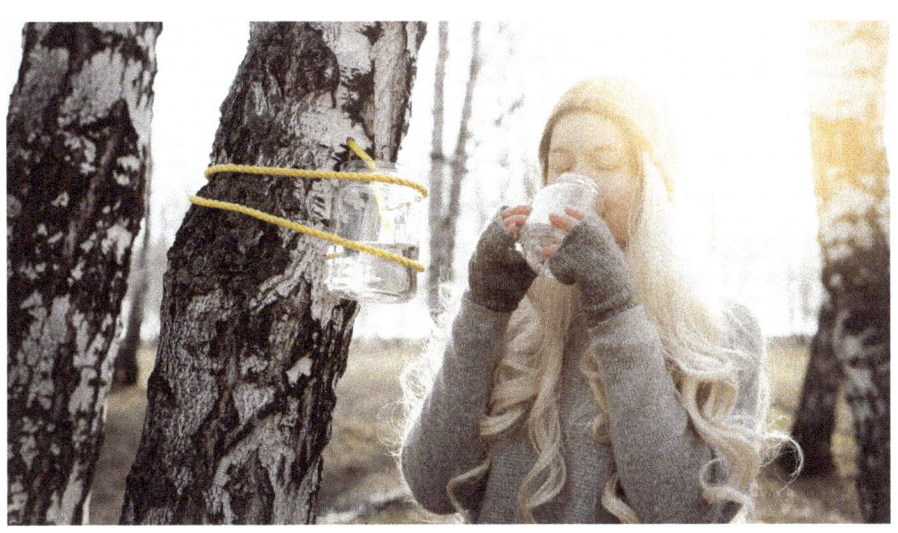

The Vikings ate with purpose. Their diet wasn't designed for convenience, it was designed for function—to survive brutal winters, to endure long voyages, to recover from physical labor, and to support fertility. And somehow, without modern nutrition labels, supplements, or macros, the Viking diet managed to be one of the most nutrient-dense and functional ways of eating humanity has ever known. Let's break it down.

FOOD FROM THE SEA AND RIVERS

Vikings relied heavily on fish and seafood for sustenance. Wild salmon, herring, trout, eel, cod, and mackerel were dietary staples. Rich in omega-3 fatty acids, protein, and minerals like iodine and selenium, these foods built strong hearts, sharp brains, and resilient immune systems. Roe (fish eggs)—a forgotten modern superfood—was considered a delicacy and is a dense source of EPA (eicosapentaenoic acid) and DHA (docosahexaenoic acid). In fact, the abundance of omega-3 fatty acids—especially DHA and EPA—is one of the most overlooked aspects of the Viking diet.

EPA and DHA are *essential* fatty acids, which means (1) our bodies don't make them, so we must consume them from our diet; and (2) these fats are essential for:

- Brain function and focus
- Mood and hormone regulation
- Inflammation control
- Immune strength
- Cardiovascular health
- Nervous system repair

Modern diets are high in omega-6 oils (corn, soy, seed oils) and low in omega-3s—which causes chronic inflammation and cellular damage. *The Modern Viking Diet* brings omega-3s back to the center of your plate, where they belong.

FOOD FROM THE LAND

Vikings absorbed important vitamins from the animals they raised—sheep, goats, pigs, and cattle. They consumed nose-to-tail—eating not just the muscle meat but also organ meats, bone marrow, and fat. Liver, heart, and kidneys were significant sources of vitamins A, D, and B12, along with iron and coenzyme Q10.

Also, fat was not feared—it was fuel. Animal fat, especially from grass-fed animals, was rendered into tallow and used in cooking. Sour milk, cheeses, and fermented whey drinks provided probiotics and healthy fats.

ANCIENT GRAINS AND ROOT VEGETABLES

Barley, rye, and oats were their primary grains. Low-gluten and high-fiber, these were prepared in porridge or flatbreads, or fermented. Vikings also foraged and cultivated root vegetables like turnips, carrots, and beets, which stored well through winter and provided slow-burning energy. Unlike modern, carb-heavy diets, the Vikings' carbohydrate sources were balanced with fat and protein, which helped stabilize blood sugar and maintain endurance.

WILD PLANTS, BERRIES, AND FERMENTED FOODS

Vikings harvested wild berries—lingonberries, bilberries, and cloudberries—that were loaded with antioxidants and natural polyphenols. They gathered nettles, dandelion, wild garlic, sorrel, and mushrooms like chanterelles and chaga, which were used for both food and medicine.

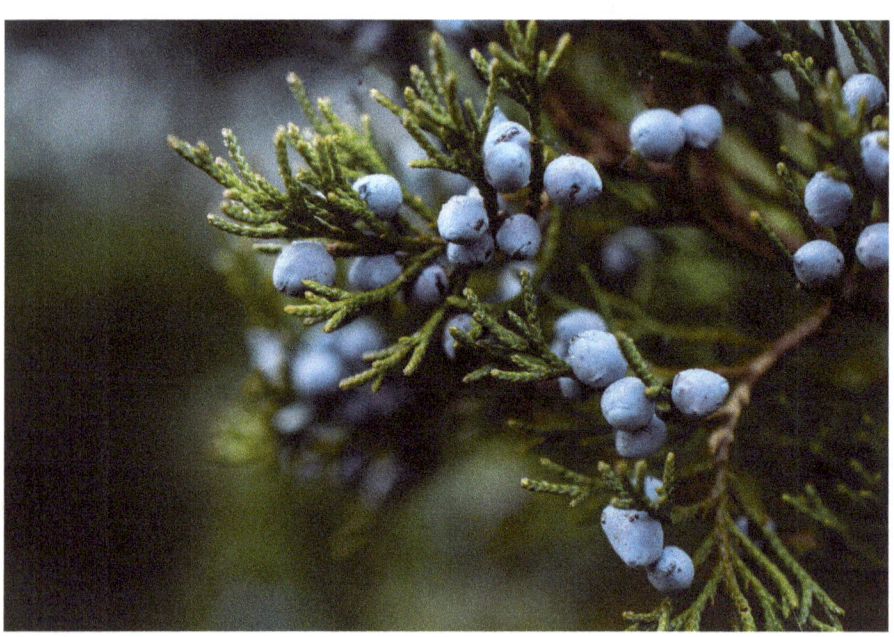

Fermentation was a way of life: Cabbage was turned into sauerkraut, fish was preserved through lactic acid fermentation, and even dairy and beverages were fermented. These foods supported gut health and immunity—long before science confirmed the importance of the microbiome.

NATURAL SWEETENERS AND BEVERAGES

Everything the Vikings drank came from nature—no chemicals, dyes, or artificial anything—and included spring water, bone broth, herbal infusions, and occasionally fermented milk. Sugar was nonexistent. Honey, the main sweetener, was used sparingly. Mead—a fermented honey beverage—was consumed during celebrations and rituals, often infused with herbs and sometimes even psychoactive mushrooms.

For the Vikings, strength wasn't only physical—it was also spiritual. They used psychoactive plants and mushrooms for ceremonies, rituals, and healing. Ritual was a part of nourishment. Food was not just fuel—it was part of a cycle of gratitude, offering, and communion with the Earth and the divine.

They ate to survive—and thrive

The Vikings were strong, not just in body—but in spirit, endurance, fertility, and recovery. They derived strength not just from what they did, but also from what they absorbed.

They didn't count calories. They ate with instinct, aligned with what their environment provided and respecting every part of the animal, plant, and process.

Their diet worked because it was:

- ✓ Anti-inflammatory
- ✓ High in omega-3 fats
- ✓ Full of pre- and probiotics
- ✓ Free from processed foods
- ✓ Rich in minerals and fat-soluble vitamins
- ✓ Aligned with nature and the seasons
- ✓ Supportive of both physical and mental resilience

MEDICINAL HERBS, PLANTS, AND TONICS OF THE VIKINGS

Food was also medicine. Ancestral plants provided strength, resilience, and healing in the Nordic world.

Nettle (Urtica dioica), often called a "super green," is one of the most nutrient-dense wild plants in Europe. Vikings used it in soups, stews, and teas—especially in the spring to rebuild energy after the long winter. Nettles are high in iron, calcium, magnesium, and vitamin C. They support blood building, adrenal function, and hair/skin health; gently detoxify the liver and kidneys; and strengthen the immune system.

Dandelion (Taraxacum officinale) is a powerhouse liver and digestive tonic. It acts as a natural diuretic to reduce water retention, balances blood sugar, provides bitter stimulation for digestion, and its leaves are rich in potassium and vitamins A and K. Vikings likely added this humble weed to broths or ate it fresh in early spring for a cleansing effect. Dandelion's bitter compounds, like sesquiterpene lactones, stimulate the liver to secrete more bile; improved bile flow is vital for the liver's role in processing and eliminating excess hormones, particularly estrogen.

Angelica root (Angelica archangelica) is a beloved Nordic herb used for protection, warming, and circulation. Vikings used it in root teas or chopped it into meat stews for warmth and resilience. The herb stimulates digestion and reduces gas/bloating, warms cold extremities (improves circulation), and helps with coughs, colds, and respiratory congestion.

Wild garlic (Allium ursinum) is a potent wild relative of garlic found in Nordic forests. Vikings ate it raw, crushed it into sauces, or added it to cooked fish and soups. Antibacterial and antifungal, wild garlic promotes heart health and circulation and supports immune defense to fight infection. It also contains sulfur compounds that aid detoxification.

Juniper berries (Juniperus communis) are antiseptic and detoxifying (especially for kidneys and the urinary tract). They stimulate digestion and bile flow, enhance respiratory health, and have a warming, slightly stimulating effect on the body. They were used both for flavoring and preserving. Vikings crushed and rubbed the berries onto meats or brewed them as a digestive tonic.

Yarrow (Achillea millefolium) is an ancient warrior herb used for healing wounds and harmonizing the body. Vikings used yarrow in teas or poultices, especially in first aid–style applications. In addition to stopping bleeding (used topically and internally), yarrow balances hormones and regulates menstrual flow, relieves fevers and colds, and supports liver and gallbladder detox.

Lovage (Levisticum officinale) is a celery-like herb that supports digestion. It is a diuretic and cleanses the kidneys, relieving bloating and fluid retention. Lovage also adds mineral-rich flavor to broths and stews and is an antioxidant and antimicrobial. It was popular in Viking kitchen gardens and for flavoring preserved foods.

Dill (Anethum graveolens) is a beloved flavoring herb and digestive aid. It soothes the stomach, relieves cramps, and is calming to the nervous system. Dill has mild antimicrobial properties and is rich in vitamin C and manganese. Vikings used dill in fermented vegetables, fish, and healing soups.

The **Chaga mushroom** (Inonotus obliquus) is a birch tree fungus revered for its immune support. Vikings likely brewed chaga as a warm decoction during long winters. Chaga is rich in antioxidants, may reduce oxidative stress, and protects DNA. It has been used to prevent cancer, reduce inflammation, and boost resilience.

Birch sap—the Viking version of a detox elixir and nature's electrolyte water—was tapped directly from birch trees during the spring. It rejuvenates the body after winter fatigue, flushes the kidneys and lymphatic system, and is naturally rich in minerals and amino acids. It tastes slightly sweet and is energizing.

Nordic berries (cloudberry, lingonberry, bilberry) were superfoods long before the term existed. The wild berries are high in vitamin C, polyphenols, and anthocyanins. They are anti-inflammatory and blood-sugar stabilizing, support brain and eye health, aid digestion, and protect gut lining. Vikings preserved the berries as jams or dried them. They ate them fresh in season with porridge or fish.

MODERN TAKEAWAY

To eat like a Viking today, focus on wild, local, unprocessed foods. Prioritize omega-3s, minerals, and organ meats, and embrace fermented and seasonal foods. Cycle between fasting and feasting, and eat with reverence and simplicity. This is how we begin to rebuild our bodies, clear our minds, and reignite our vitality—one meal at a time. Turn to page 15 for an in-depth look at these and the other core principles.

CORE PRINCIPLES

Heal like your ancestors would—wild, whole, and wise.

To thrive today, we must take the wisdom of the old ways and blend it with the best of modern nutrition science—not trends, not fads, but timeless principles rooted in both nature and science—what actually works to build a strong, clear, resilient body. Below are the nine core principles of the Viking diet, expanded for today's world.

#1: EAT REAL, WHOLE, WILD FOOD

Before superfoods, macros, or calorie counting, there was only one kind of food: real food. Food that grew wild, swam free, sprouted from fertile earth, and nourished entire civilizations. The Vikings didn't eat ultra-processed snacks, seed oils, or synthetic additives. They didn't need labels like *organic* or *pasture-raised*—because everything was. They ate food that was alive. This is the foundation of your health. If the body is built from what you feed it, then real food creates real strength.

Real food is grown or raised naturally, without chemicals; recognizable by your ancestors; full of color, texture, enzymes, and minerals; and minimally processed or cooked in traditional ways (steamed, roasted, fermented, dried).

Real food is not made in a lab; packaged in plastic with thirty ingredients; full of preservatives, flavor enhancers, or synthetic vitamins; stripped of fiber, enzymes, and life force. If it wouldn't grow, swim, or walk in the wild—or rot naturally in a week—it's not real food.

Real food matters now more than ever. Your body is exposed to thousands of modern toxins daily: plastics, microplastics, pesticides, industrial oils, fake flavorings, emulsifiers, and synthetic "nutrients" the body doesn't recognize. These ingredients confuse your cells, inflame your gut, clog your liver, and disrupt your hormones.

Real food, on the other hand:

- ✓ Builds healthy tissue
- ✓ Repairs the gut lining
- ✓ Nourishes the mitochondria
- ✓ Balances blood sugar and insulin
- ✓ Lowers inflammation and oxidative stress
- ✓ Brings you back to your natural energy and mental clarity

Real food isn't a diet. It's your birthright. Remember: Your cells are rebuilding themselves every second of every day. The quality of what you eat determines what you're made of. Eat like your ancestors—eat to become unbreakable: Eat food that looks (and smells) like food. Prioritize quality over quantity. Choose wild, local, and organic when possible. Cook like a Viking—slow, simple, seasonal—and eat with intention, not distraction.

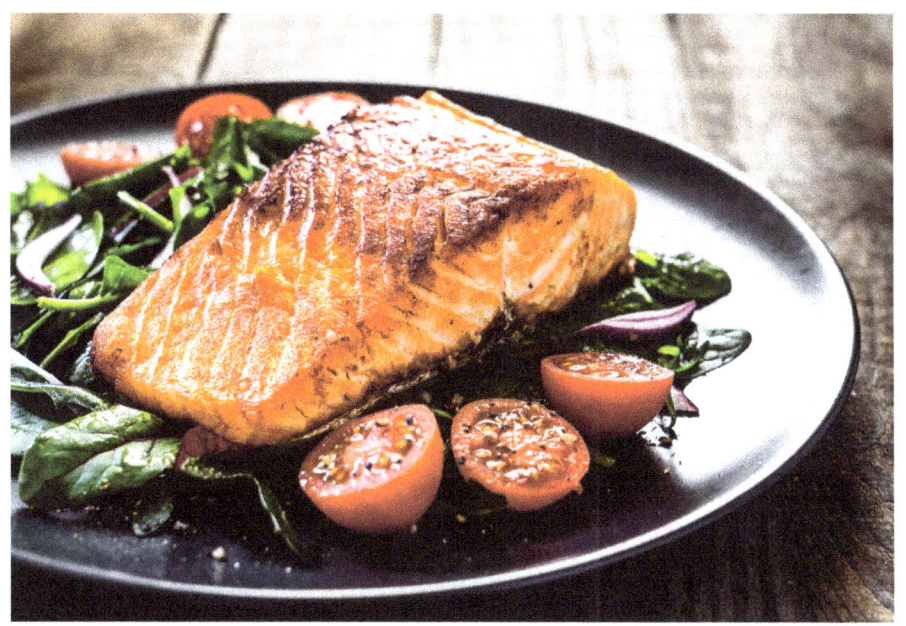

#2: NOURISH YOUR CELLS WITH OMEGA-3S—THE FOUNDATION OF HEALTH

Your body is made up of around 37 trillion cells, and every one of those cells is wrapped in a membrane made of fat. The health, flexibility, and intelligence of that membrane determines everything about how your body functions. Omega-3 fatty acids—especially EPA and DHA, which only come from the ocean (either algae or fish)—are the very fats your body uses to build those membranes.

DHA makes up over 90 percent of the omega-3 fats in the brain—the synaptic connections that allow thinking, memory, and emotion, and the gray matter involved in reasoning and cognition—and over 60 percent of the retina in your eyes. Therefore, DHA is essential for mental clarity and vision health.

Omega-3s protect you from:

- Cardiovascular disease
- Depression, anxiety, and cognitive decline
- ADHD and autism spectrum disorders
- Autoimmune conditions like rheumatoid arthritis and lupus
- Diabetes and insulin resistance
- Chronic skin issues like eczema and psoriasis
- Macular degeneration and vision loss

A study published in *The Journal of Clinical Lipidology* found that higher blood levels of omega-3s were associated with up to a 90 percent lower risk of sudden cardiac death. Research in *The Journal of the American College of Cardiology* shows EPA and DHA reduce triglycerides, stabilize heart rhythms, lower blood pressure, and prevent plaque buildup. *The Lancet Neurology* linked DHA to improved cognition and reduced risk of Alzheimer's disease. In one study, low DHA levels were associated with a measurable shrinkage of brain volume over time.

WHEN YOU'RE DEFICIENT

Omega-3s are the foundation of cellular health, controlling inflammation at the molecular level. Without them, your cells become stiff, inflamed, and dysfunctional—and your body can't:

- Repair damaged cells
- Produce optimal hormones

- Regulate immunity
- Protect your brain from degeneration
- Maintain mood stability and emotional regulation
- Support fetal and childhood development

Research has found that inflammatory diseases are all tied to imbalanced omega-6:omega-3 ratios. The ideal ratio is 1:1 or 2:1. Most Americans eat at a ratio of 20:1 or higher, tipping the body toward chronic inflammation. This imbalance is not just unhealthy, it's dangerous—but it *is* reversible.

How did we become so deficient? To start, industrial farming eliminated omega-3–rich grasses from animals' diets. Nowadays, fish is often farm-raised and lower in omega-3s. Plant oils (canola, corn, soy) dominate processed food, which also pushes omega-6 sky-high. The modern diet is anti-DHA—and our chronic disease burden proves it.

To reclaim your cellular strength, your shopping list should be filled with today's top omega-3 sources:

- Wild-caught salmon, sardines, anchovies
- Cod liver oil (also gives you vitamins A and D in synergy)
- Pasture-raised eggs (especially omega-3 enriched)
- Algae oil, for plant-based, environmentally conscious, or if you want a super pure source

---
Tip: Try to avoid cheap brands with oxidized oils or fillers.

Think of omega-3s as the insulation for your body's electrical wires. Without them, signals are scrambled and systems short-circuit. They are your number-one daily nonnegotiable. If you only take one supplement, let it be omega-3s. You are only as healthy as your cell membranes. And your membranes are built from what you eat.

#3: MASTER BLOOD SUGAR— THE FOUNDATION OF VITALITY

If there were one thread woven through nearly every modern disease, it would be dysregulated blood sugar. From fatigue to brain fog, belly fat to mood swings, high blood pressure to early cognitive decline—the root often traces back to imbalances in how our body processes glucose. Blood sugar regulation is not just a concern for diabetics. It is central to human biology and evolution, and understanding it is crucial for reclaiming health in our sugar-saturated, stress-driven modern world.

Blood sugar is the amount of glucose circulating in your bloodstream at any given time. It is the primary fuel for your brain, your muscles, and every cell in your body. However, too much or too little can cause serious harm.

After you eat, carbohydrates are broken down into glucose. In response, your pancreas releases insulin, a hormone that encourages glucose to enter your cells to be used or stored for later. In an ideal world, your body maintains tight control over this process—blood sugar rises moderately after meals, insulin brings it back down smoothly, and energy is steady throughout the day. But that's not the world we live in anymore.

The modern crisis is ricocheting glucose. Thanks to ultra-processed foods, chronic stress, artificial light exposure, poor sleep, and constant snacking, most people today are unknowingly riding a blood sugar roller-coaster—spiking high, crashing low, and repeating the cycle all day long. This metabolic chaos leads to:

- Insulin resistance—Your cells stop responding to insulin, so your body has to pump out more and more. Eventually, blood sugar stays elevated, paving the path toward pre-diabetes and type 2 diabetes.
- Weight gain—especially around the belly, due to increased insulin (a fat-storage hormone)
- Energy crashes and cravings—Glucose highs feel good for a short time, but they lead to crashes that make you crave more sugar or caffeine.
- Hormonal havoc—Insulin imbalances affect cortisol, estrogen, testosterone, and thyroid hormones, and throw your entire endocrine system off balance.
- Accelerated aging—Chronically high blood sugar damages proteins in your body through a process called glycation, contributing to wrinkles, stiff joints, cataracts, and even Alzheimer's (now dubbed *type 3 diabetes*).

A 2018 study in *The Lancet* linked poor blood sugar regulation to increased risk of cardiovascular disease, even in people without diabetes. Chronically elevated glucose also leads to oxidative stress, damaging your mitochondria—the very engines of your cells. Research also shows that even brief glucose spikes after meals impair cognitive function and raise inflammatory markers like C-reactive protein (CRP).

REGULATE BLOOD SUGAR NATURALLY—
THE VIKING WAY

Our ancestors consumed whole foods that kept their blood sugar in balance—wild meats, fish, fermented vegetables, tubers, nuts, and berries. They didn't have access to refined flour, corn syrup, or constant food availability. Meals were spaced apart. Fasting was natural. Physical activity was constant. When they did eat carbohydrates (like rye bread or root vegetables), they were always paired with fiber, fat, and protein—which slowed glucose absorption and prevented spikes. This is the biological norm; our genes are still wired for that lifestyle.

Here's how you can bring blood sugar into balance today, Viking-style:

- Build your plate right. Prioritize protein first at every meal (wild fish, grass-fed meat, legumes). Add healthy fats like olive oil, wild salmon, or flax—omega-3s. Choose slow carbs—roots, berries, and soaked grains—and avoid naked carbs (e.g., just fruit or crackers without protein/fat). Bitter greens and sour ferments—think, arugula, sauerkraut, and vinegar-based dressings—also improve insulin sensitivity and promote digestive enzyme release.
- Constant grazing keeps insulin elevated. Try to space out your meals, giving 4–5 hrs. between eating. And invest in some glucose-supporting nutrients, like chromium and magnesium, to help regulate insulin. Herbs like berberine, cinnamon, and gymnema also improve glucose metabolism.

- Other than your intake, what else can you do? Exercise! Even a 10-minute walk after meals can lower glucose spikes by 20–30 percent, according to studies.
- Balance your cortisol: Chronic stress raises blood sugar. Incorporate breath work, acupuncture, nature time, or adaptogens like reishi or holy basil.
- Consider using a continuous glucose monitor (CGM) for data-driven feedback if needed.

When your blood sugar is steady, your mood stabilizes, your brain sharpens, your hormones harmonize, and your cravings dissolve. You tap into a state of calm vitality that feels like your body is finally working *with* you—not against you. The modern world pushes us into chaos. But metabolic stability is your superpower—and your first defense against aging, inflammation, and burnout. Eat like a Viking, live like a sage, and keep your blood sugar steady. Your entire body will thank you!

EXAMPLE MEAL PLAN

Below is a plan that is glucose-stabilizing and deeply nourishing.

OPTIONAL PRE-BREAKFAST RITUAL

Drink 16 ounces of warm lemon water with a pinch of sea salt to hydrate and support adrenal balance. Follow up with some gentle movement or breath work to activate the parasympathetic nervous system.

BREAKFAST (8–9 A.M.)

Wild Protein Bowl

2 pasture-raised eggs (or tempeh if vegan) sautéed in ghee or olive oil
½ avocado, sliced
½ cup sautéed bitter greens (dandelion, kale, or arugula)
2 tbsp. fermented vegetables (sauerkraut or kimchi)
Sprinkle of hemp or flaxseeds
Herbal tea: nettle and cinnamon infusion (supports blood sugar and adrenal health)
Why it works: healthy fats + fiber + protein + bitter greens = no glucose spike, longer satiety, better hormone balance

LUNCH (12–1 P.M.)

Nordic Power Salad

Wild-caught salmon or grilled elk strips
Base of mixed greens (arugula, watercress, spinach)
Roasted beets or parsnips (cooled; resistant starch supports the microbiome.)
Pickled red onions and capers
Olive oil and apple cider vinegar dressing
Side: 1 slice of seed-based crispbread (see Viking Flatbread recipe, page 190)
Why it works: balanced macronutrients, added fermented and bitter foods, no hidden sugars, fiber-rich

AFTERNOON STABILIZER (3–4 P.M.)

Chaga Chai Elixir

Brewed chaga tea with unsweetened coconut or almond milk
Spices: cinnamon, cardamom, and a touch of clove
Optional: Add 1 tsp. coconut oil or MCT oil for brain and blood sugar support.
Snack (only if needed): 1 small handful of walnuts and 1 Brazil nut OR a boiled egg with turmeric sea salt
Why it works: Adaptogens like chaga balance cortisol; healthy fat prevents crashes.

DINNER (5:30–6:30 P.M.)

Herb-Infused Broth Bowl

Base: homemade bone broth or mineral broth
Add-ins: chopped cabbage, nettles, shiitake mushrooms, garlic, leeks
Protein: shredded pasture-raised chicken or tempeh
Topped with: a drizzle of flax or hemp oil and fresh parsley and dulse flakes
Side: lightly sautéed bitter greens with lemon and olive oil
Why it works: light, easy to digest, nutrient-dense, and blood sugar–neutral to prepare for deep sleep

EVENING RITUAL (7–8 P.M.)

Drink a magnesium-rich tea (chamomile, lemon balm, or hibiscus and cinnamon).
Optional: Drink one teaspoon of apple cider vinegar in water before bed to help with overnight glucose control.

#4: CYCLE FASTING AND FEASTING TO ACTIVATE AUTOPHAGY FOR LONGEVITY

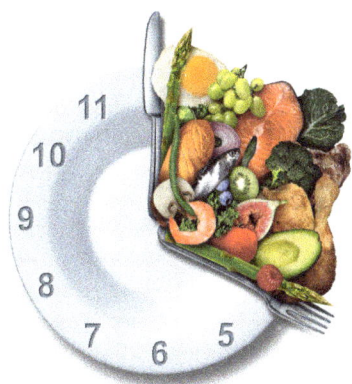

Vikings didn't snack all day. They feasted when food was abundant, and fasted when it was not. They fasted because they had to—when the hunt failed, when the seas were rough, or during the long, cold Nordic winters. That rhythm wasn't a diet—it was nature's design. They adapted. They became sharper, stronger, more resilient. This rhythm created *metabolic flexibility*—the ability to burn both sugar and fat for fuel.

Today, we've lost that rhythm. We eat constantly, never giving our bodies the chance to reset, detox, or shift into deep healing mode. That's where strategic fasting comes in.

Modern fasting rhythms:

- ✓ Practice intermittent fasting (12–16 hrs. overnight).
- ✓ Eat two to three meals per day, no snacks.
- ✓ Seasonal fasts during spring and fall
- ✓ Occasional 24-hr. resets or broth/juice days

Fasting gives your body a break from digestion so it can focus on cell repair, inflammation control, hormone regulation, and fat burning. It activates autophagy—a natural cleanup process that clears out damaged cells. Think of it like an internal cleanse, every single day.

Fasting isn't deprivation. It's sacred rest. It's strategic—and it's built into your DNA. Today, fasting is no longer a survival necessity, but it's still one of the most powerful health tools you can use to awaken cellular repair, burn fat, and reclaim metabolic freedom.

During a fast:

- Insulin levels drop, allowing fat burning to begin.
- Human growth hormone (HGH) increases, supporting muscle retention and anti-aging.
- Autophagy kicks in—your cells clean up old, damaged parts.
- Inflammation decreases.
- Mental clarity improves.
- Digestion resets.
- Your mitochondria (energy factories) become more efficient.

What Happens in the Body During a Fast?	
Hours Fasted	What Happens
8–12 hrs	Blood sugar and insulin drop.
12–16 hrs	Fat burning begins.

16–24 hrs	Human growth hormone surges.
24–36 hrs	Autophagy and deep repair begin.
36–72 hrs	Stem cell regeneration—full reset.

TYPES OF FASTING

What follows are the most powerful and popular fasting styles, each with their unique benefits.

INTERMITTENT FASTING (TIME-RESTRICTED EATING)

How it works: You fast for 14–20 hrs. and eat during a window of 4–10 hrs.

Popular ratios:
- 16:8 (fast 16 hrs., eat within 8 hrs.)
- 18:6 or 20:4 for more intensity
- Eat dinner early, skip breakfast, break your fast with protein + fat + fiber
- Benefits:
- Blood sugar balance
- Fat loss without calorie counting
- Better energy and mood
- Improved digestion
- Reduces snacking and cravings

Tip: Most people thrive on 16:8 fasting a few days a week.

24-HR. FAST (1–2X PER WEEK)

How it works: Eat dinner, then don't eat again until the next day's dinner.

Benefits:
- » Deep insulin sensitivity reset
- » Stimulates autophagy
- » Improves gut healing
- » Clears mental fog and boosts focus

Tips: Stay hydrated, sip herbal tea, and use electrolytes if needed. Ideal to pair with a day of rest, nature, or spiritual practice.

EXTENDED FASTS: 36–72 HRS.

How it works: Fast for two to three days on water, herbal tea, and electrolytes.

Benefits:
- » Profound cellular repair
- » Massive autophagy and stem cell activation
- » Detox of senescent (old, damaged) cells

» Powerful for metabolic reset, autoimmune flares, and gut repair

Tips: This is not for beginners. Always prepare with clean eating before and after. Consult a practitioner if dealing with chronic illness or medication.

OTHER FASTING STYLES YOU CAN EXPLORE

Fat Fasting: Consume only healthy fats (e.g., MCT oil, ghee, avocados) for a few days to stimulate ketosis.

Bone Broth Fast: Healing for the gut, this fast adds minerals and collagen, and keeps blood sugar stable.

Juice Fast: This is a more traditional variation, but higher in sugar. It is best with greens, ginger, and lemon.

Spiritual Fast: Intentionally abstaining from something desirable, often food, the primary purpose of this fast is to seek God, deepen spiritual awareness, and/or address a specific spiritual need.

WHAT CAN YOU HAVE DURING A FAST?

The goal is to keep insulin low and avoid triggering digestion so your body can stay in a fat-burning, autophagy-boosting state. Science shows that pure water, herbal teas, black coffee, and minerals generally do *not* break a fast and can actually enhance the benefits—like improved mental clarity, mitochondrial health, and cellular cleanup. Black coffee (without sweeteners or milk) has been shown to support fat metabolism and autophagy, thanks to its polyphenols and caffeine. However, adding milk or cream (even plant-based) introduces calories and carbohydrates, which can raise insulin and technically break the fast.

The stricter your fasting goals (e.g., deep autophagy or hormone reset), the cleaner your fast should be. That said, a small amount of fat (like MCT oil or ghee) may be acceptable in certain fasting styles like fat fasting or modified intermittent fasting, especially if it helps with adherence or mental focus. For best results during a fast, stick to the following:

- Water (filtered, mineral, or with lemon slice—no pulp)
- Herbal teas (nettle, chamomile, mint, tulsi, rooibos—unsweetened)
- Black coffee (organic, no sugar or milk)
- Minerals and electrolytes (like sea salt, magnesium drops)
- Apple cider vinegar (1 tsp. in water—may support blood sugar)
- Sparkling water (no sweeteners)
- Optional in modified fasts: 1 tsp. MCT oil, coconut oil, or ghee (for brain fuel)

AVOID DURING A FAST

- × Milk or cream (even almond or coconut)
- × Sweeteners (even stevia or monk fruit if you're fasting for insulin sensitivity or gut healing)

- ✗ Broths (unless doing a bone broth fast or using it to break the fast)
- ✗ Anything with calories, protein, or carbs

Think of fasting as a cellular reset—keep it clean, keep it simple, and let your body do what it was designed to do: heal itself. It's also important to remember that fasting isn't for everyone. If you're pregnant, breastfeeding, underweight, or dealing with chronic fatigue or thyroid issues—approach fasting gently or avoid extended fasts. And women may need to fast differently altogether.

Fasting is a powerful longevity tool—one that cleanses the body, sharpens the mind, and awakens ancient survival pathways. Just as the Vikings tailored their strategies to the season, the terrain, and the individual, fasting must also be adapted to the person. What fuels vitality for one body might drain it in another. This is especially true when we consider the unique physiology of women, whose hormonal rhythms require a different, more nuanced approach than the "one-size-fits-all" fasting advice often promoted today.

THE VIKING WOMAN'S WAY: FLOW, NOT FORCE

In the Viking tradition, women were warriors and healers—intuitive, powerful, and connected to nature's rhythms. Fasting, when done correctly, restores rhythm, resets your metabolism, and amplifies clarity. But for women, it must be done in harmony with the female cycle—not in defiance of it.

What works for men (or even postmenopausal women) can backfire for women in their reproductive years—especially if fasting is done too aggressively. Female bodies are hormonally dynamic and highly attuned to stress, so prolonged calorie restriction can trigger anxiety, fatigue, hair loss, thyroid imbalance, and menstrual disruptions. Red flags include losing your period, cold hands and feet, hair thinning, racing thoughts, poor sleep or waking at 3 a.m., and intense evening cravings for sugar or carbs. These aren't signs of discipline—they're your body's way of saying, "This feels like a threat." Always listen first, adjust with care, and let your fasting rhythm support your biology—not fight it.

So how do we fast in a way that honors female physiology, supports long-term health, and taps into the ancient wisdom of metabolic flexibility? The answer lies in timing, rhythm, and intuition. A woman's body is designed to create life, and it's constantly assessing: "Is it safe to reproduce?" Prolonged fasting or extreme caloric restriction can send the wrong signal: "This is not a safe time." This is especially true during certain phases of the menstrual cycle when estrogen or progesterone are elevated—times when the body naturally increases metabolic demands and needs more nourishment, not less.

In the follicular phase (menstruation to ovulation), rising estrogen makes the body more resilient to fasting, so longer windows may feel easier. But in the luteal phase (after ovulation), progesterone dominance increases calorie needs, speeds up metabolism, and heightens sensitivity to stress, making shorter fasts or more balanced meals the wiser choice. The key? Cycle-sync your fasting so it works with your biology—not against it. Let's break the cycle down into fasting-friendly (and fasting-cautious) phases:

Week 1—Menstrual (Days 1–5)

Best fasting style: Gentle or none
Why: Your body is shedding the uterine lining, hormones

are low, and energy is lower. This is a time for nourishment and rest.

Tip: Try 12-hr. overnight fasts only, with broth, warming foods, and minerals.

Week 2—Follicular (Days 6–13)

Best fasting style: Moderate fasting works beautifully here.
Why: Estrogen is rising, and your body is more insulin-sensitive. Energy and brain clarity increase.

Tip: Try 14-to-16-hour fasts a few days per week. You'll likely feel sharp and light. This is a great time for deeper work, strength training, or fat-burning.

Week 3—Ovulation and Early Luteal (Days 14–21)

Best fasting style: Pull back slightly.
Why: Estrogen peaks, then starts to drop. Progesterone begins to rise (especially post-ovulation), which increases appetite and insulin resistance slightly.

Tips: Try 13-to-15-hour fasts max. Don't fast aggressively. Prioritize fiber and complex carbs to support progesterone production.

Week 4—Late Luteal/PMS (Days 22-28)

Best fasting style: Gentle, nourishing, no extended fasts
Why: Progesterone peaks, then drops. Your body is more sensitive to stress. This is the most important week to back off fasting, caffeine, and extreme workouts.

Tips: Try 12-hour circadian fasts only. Think grounding meals, magnesium-rich foods, root veggies, and healthy carbs.

POSTMENOPAUSAL

Once you're no longer cycling monthly, fasting becomes more stable and flexible. You can ease into longer intermittent fasting (16:8, 18:6) and even experiment with 24-hour fasts or weekly autophagy resets, as long as you're well-nourished and not under chronic stress. Think of postmenopausal fasting as a return to your warrior archetype—your body is no longer conserving energy for reproduction and is more resilient to metabolic shifts.

TYPES OF FASTS FOR WOMEN AND WHEN TO USE THEM

- Circadian Fast: 12-13 hours—a daily gentle baseline for all women
- Intermittent Fast: 14-16 hours—during follicular phase or post-menopause

- 24-Hr. Reset Fast: Once per week—optional for autophagy in healthy women
- Autophagy Cleanse: 36–48 hours—monthly or quarterly, but only if experienced and hormonally stable

The most powerful fast is the one that leaves you feeling energized, balanced, and resilient—not depleted. Honor your design. Fast like a goddess. Feast like a queen. And trust your body's sacred timing.

FASTING-SUPPORTIVE TOOLS FOR WOMEN

- Herbs for blood sugar and stress: cinnamon, holy basil, berberine, nettle, licorice root
- Minerals: magnesium, potassium, sea salt in morning water (especially for mood and energy)
- Gentle movement: walking, rebounding, yoga during fasts
- Break the fast with protein and fat first (eggs, avocado, wild fish), then add veggies or carbs second.
- Support hormones: seed cycling, omega-3s, B vitamins, adaptogens like maca or ashwagandha. Seed cycling involves eating different types of seeds at different phases of the menstrual cycle to support hormonal balance. Eat flax and pumpkin seeds during the follicular phase for estrogen production and balance. Eat sesame and sunflower seeds during the luteal phase for progesterone production and to help regulate estrogen levels.

CYCLE-SYNCED FASTING DAY EXAMPLE (FOLLICULAR PHASE)

This is ideal for days six through thirteen of the menstrual cycle (or anytime for postmenopausal women). Target fast: 16:8 (16 hours fasting/8 hours eating window).

MORNING (FASTING WINDOW) | 7:00–11:00 A.M.

Hydration and hormone support: no calories, but plenty of nourishment

Warm lemon water (16 oz.) and pinch of sea salt

Optional: herbal tea (nettle, holy basil, or cinnamon)
1 scoop of minerals or electrolytes in water

Optional light movement: 20-minute walk, yoga flow, breath work, or rebounding

Mental clarity tools: journaling, sunlight exposure, meditation

BREAK THE FAST (MEAL #1) | 11:00 A.M.

Omega-Powered Protein Plate

2 pasture-raised eggs (soft-boiled or poached)
¼ avocado
Sautéed arugula or dandelion greens in olive oil
2 tbsp. fermented veggies (sauerkraut or kimchi)
Sprinkle of hemp seeds and sea salt

Herbal drink: hibiscus and cinnamon tea

Why it works: Protein and fat help break the fast gently. Bitter greens stimulate bile, digestion, and hormone support. Ferments improve insulin sensitivity.

MID-DAY NOURISHMENT (MEAL #2) | 3:00 P.M.

Viking Spring Bowl

Grilled wild salmon or lentil patties
Baby greens and roasted beets
Chopped cucumber, dill, lemon, olive oil
Topped with: pumpkin seeds and seaweed flakes
½ small roasted sweet potato (cooled = resistant starch)

Drink: chaga tea with coconut milk, cinnamon, cardamom

Why it works: This nourishing, balanced meal ends your eating window with minerals, slow carbs, omega-3s, and glucose-buffering fiber—perfect for luteinizing hormone and brain health support.

EVENING (FASTING RESUMES) | 7:00 P.M. ONWARD

No food

Drink warm herbal tea: chamomile, lemon balm, or tulsi. Take magnesium or mineral support before bed.

Optional: journaling, grounding, castor oil pack, or gentle yin yoga

#5: FOCUS ON BITTER, FERMENTED, AND WILD FOODS—THE FORGOTTEN HEALERS FOR GUT AND IMMUNE SYSTEM SUPPORT

Vikings didn't eat for comfort. They ate for resilience, survival, and strength. That's why their diet was naturally filled with bitter herbs, fermented vegetables, and wild plants—foods that modern people have nearly forgotten. Most of the modern Western diet is dominated by sweet and salty flavors—often ultra-processed and stripped of real nutrition. But true health requires balance—and bitter, sour (fermented), and even pungent foods play a vital role in stimulating digestion, detoxification, and microbiome diversity. These aren't just trendy add-ons. They're the missing link in most modern diets—and it's time to reclaim them.

These three categories—bitter, fermented, and wild—stimulate different systems in the body that are essential for daily detox, gut health, and metabolic balance. These foods are more than just trends or ancient relics—they are the sacred, healing forces that modern diets have forgotten. In Chinese medicine, they are seen as essential to nourishing our core vitality, clearing heat, draining dampness, and replenishing the organs that govern longevity—especially the kidneys, liver, and spleen.

BITTERS

In Chinese medicine, bitter is the flavor that nourishes the heart and supports the kidneys—our core longevity organs responsible for vitality, hormonal balance, and deep constitutional strength. Yet, in today's Western diet, bitter foods are nearly extinct—replaced by sweet, salty, and processed flavors that overstimulate and deplete the body. Bitters act as a powerful digestive tonic, helping to stimulate bile flow, detoxify the liver, regulate blood sugar, and calm inflammation. They also strengthen the parasympathetic (rest-and-digest) nervous system. If we want to age gracefully, preserve our energy, and avoid disease, we must reclaim bitter foods as a daily ritual of resilience.

Some popular bitters:
- ✓ Dandelion roots or leaves
- ✓ Artichoke leaves
- ✓ Gentian roots
- ✓ Arugula, radicchio
- ✓ Bitter melons
- ✓ Lemon peels or grapefruit rinds

Benefits:
- Stimulate bile production (crucial for fat digestion and liver detox)
- Awaken digestive enzymes
- Support pancreas, liver, and gallbladder function
- Help regulate appetite and cravings
- Aid in blood sugar control
- Promote smooth bowel movements

It is best to eat bitters in the morning or midday when digestive fire (yang) is rising—ideally before meals (as a tonic or in salads). This is especially powerful during spring, the season of the liver and renewal.

LONGEVITY BITTERS SHOT— A SIMPLE DAILY TONIC RECIPE

Ingredients:
1 tbsp. raw apple cider vinegar
Juice of ½ lemon
2 slices fresh ginger
3 dandelion or arugula leaves (muddled or juiced if desired)
Optional: pinch of sea salt and 1 tsp. aloe vera juice

Instructions: Mix in a small glass and drink before your biggest meal of the day.

Tip: Keep a small jar pre-mixed in the fridge for two to three days. Drink it like a tonic shot or dilute in warm water as a tea.

FERMENTED FOODS

Over 70 percent of your immune system lives in your gut, and the health of that system depends largely on your microbiome—the trillions of beneficial bacteria that help you digest food, produce nutrients, and protect against invaders. Fermented foods are one of the most powerful (and ancient) ways to support this internal ecosystem. They provide natural probiotics, enhance nutrient absorption, reduce inflammation, and help regulate metabolism and mood. Unfortunately, most modern diets are sterile and lifeless, missing these essential microbial allies. Reintroducing ferments such as the ones below helps restore balance and build a resilient body from the inside out:

- Sauerkraut
- Kimchi
- Kefir or yogurt (goat's milk or coconut)
- Beet kvass
- Fermented fish (gravlax)
- Miso or fermented garlic

Benefits:
- Rebuild the gut microbiome with beneficial bacteria
- Improve nutrient absorption, especially B vitamins and minerals
- Help seal and restore the gut lining
- Produce natural, short-chain fatty acids and vitamin K2
- Reduce bloating, constipation, and food sensitivity symptoms
- Boost mood and immune response through the gut-brain axis

Eat fermented foods in small amounts daily with meals. They can be consumed with breakfast (e.g., sauerkraut with eggs), lunch (beet kvass), or dinner (fermented vegetables). They are especially helpful after illness, antibiotic use, or periods of stress, and most supportive during late summer and fall, times of digestion and transition.

BEET KVASS RECIPE—A GUT-HEALING VIKING TONIC

Ingredients:
2–3 medium organic beets (peeled and chopped into cubes)
1 tablespoon sea salt (non-iodized)
Filtered water to fill a one-quart jar
Optional: 1 clove garlic, 3 slices fresh ginger, or 1 tablespoon caraway seeds for added flavor

Instructions: Place beets (and optional flavorings) into a clean glass jar. Add salt and fill the jar with filtered water, leaving about one inch at the top. Stir or shake gently to dissolve the salt. Cover loosely with a lid or cloth and let sit at room temperature for three to five days. Once slightly sour and earthy in taste, strain into a clean jar and refrigerate. Drink 2–4 oz. daily before meals to support digestion, liver function, and microbiome balance.

WILD FOODS

Wild foods are some of the most nutrient-dense, antioxidant-rich, and energetically potent plants on the planet. Unlike cultivated produce, which has been bred for sweetness and shelf life, wild foods grow in harsh, untamed environments—developing an incredible concentration of phytonutrients, minerals, bitter compounds, and protective antioxidants. In Chinese medicine, they are seen as *Jing* tonics—supporting primal vitality and resilience. Modern research confirms they're often higher in polyphenols, magnesium, and immune-modulating compounds than store-bought vegetables. Regularly including the wild foods below helps build strength, detoxify the body, reduce inflammation, and reconnect us to the rhythms of nature:

- Nettle, sorrel, purslane, chickweed
- Wild garlic (ramsons)
- Chaga or reishi mushrooms
- Bilberries, lingonberries
- Seaweed (dulse, kelp)

Benefits:
- Contain higher nutrient density than cultivated crops
- Rich in polyphenols, antioxidants, and trace minerals
- Often more bitter, fibrous, and cleansing to the system
- Build resilience in the body—just like the wild foods survived harsh climates, they help you adapt too.
- Reconnect you to nature's intelligence

You should eat wild foods as often as available—rotate them with the seasons. They are great in spring and summer, when wild greens are abundant and cleansing, and especially beneficial during times of fatigue, stagnation, or when reconnecting to nature is needed. You may notice how easy it is to combine wild foods into meals twice or thrice a week as pestos, teas, soups, or blended into broths and smoothies.

WILD GREENS PESTO— THE VIKING SUPERFOOD SPREAD

Ingredients:
1 cup fresh wild greens (e.g., dandelion leaves, nettles, chickweed, lamb's quarters)
½ cup fresh parsley or basil (to balance bitterness)
¼ cup raw pumpkin seeds or walnuts
1–2 garlic cloves
Juice of ½ lemon
½ cup olive oil
Sea salt to taste

Instructions: If using nettles, blanch quickly in hot water to remove sting. Add all ingredients to a food processor or blender and pulse until smooth. Taste and adjust salt or lemon as needed. Spread on toast or crackers, mix into soups or salad dressings, or serve as a nutrient-dense dip.

Tip: This pesto is loaded with magnesium, iron, chlorophyll, and detoxifying bitter compounds—making it an easy daily upgrade for energy, blood building, and immune strength.

BRING THE FORGOTTEN TRINITY INTO YOUR DAILY RHYTHM

Bitter, fermented, and wild foods connect us back to nature—raw, unpredictable, and wise. They speak the language of resilience. They whisper to the gut, the immune system, and the mitochondria: "Wake up. Detox. Adapt. Thrive." That's why you should incorporate at least one food from each category daily. For example:

- Morning: lemon and bitter tonic
- Midday: salad with wild greens and fermented kraut
- Evening: herbal broth with wild herbs or a shot of beet kvass

This is real functional nutrition—where every bite becomes medicine, and every day becomes a ritual of renewal. The farther we drift from wild, bitter, and fermented, the more inflamed, imbalanced, and disconnected we become. But when we bring them back onto our plate, even in small amounts, the body remembers. Let your food awaken your inner healer. Let your kitchen become your apothecary. And let your vitality become unshakable.

#6: LET FOOD BE YOUR MEDICINE

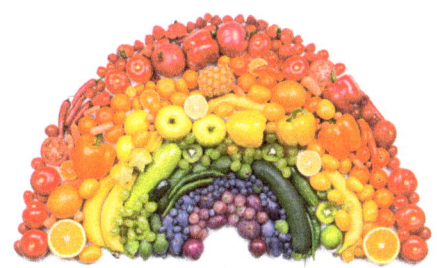

Food is not just fuel. It's information. It's construction material. It's medicine—or it's poison. Every bite you take is building or breaking you, either moving you closer to health or pulling you further into dysfunction. There is no neutral food. Everything you eat either feeds inflammation or fights it. It either burdens your liver or frees it. It clouds your mind or sharpens it. What you eat becomes your blood, your skin, your brain, your children. Let that sink in.

You become what you absorb, what you metabolize, and what your cells build themselves from. Food becomes you. The fats in your cell membranes, the neurotransmitters in your brain, the hormones that drive your energy, libido, and focus, the immune cells that defend your body—they are all built from what you eat.

When you eat processed food—chemical-laden, nutrient-empty, lifeless—you become foggy, bloated, tired, irritable, and inflamed. When you eat real food—wild, fermented, bitter, colorful—you become clear, grounded, strong, energized, and focused.

What you eat affects everything:

- Your productivity (brain clarity, energy, focus)
- Your mood (dopamine, serotonin, GABA all require amino acids and cofactors from food)

- Your motivation and drive
- Your emotions and resilience
- Your recovery from stress or illness
- Your ability to connect with others and feel joy

You literally become a different version of yourself depending on what's on your plate.

Food is a daily choice to heal or harm. Imagine this: Every bite is either a deposit or a withdrawal from your health account. It's not about perfection—it's about patterns. It's about waking up to what you're choosing every day, multiple times a day. Even small shifts (like replacing a processed snack with wild blueberries, or drinking herbal tea instead of soda) create compound benefits over time. Your body is always listening. Every bite is a message.

FOOD IS INFORMATION

Modern nutrition often reduces food to numbers: calories, carbs, fats, and proteins. But in reality, food is code. It is the language your cells speak. Every bite you take delivers biochemical signals that either promote healing or provoke harm.

In Viking and other ancient cultures, food was never separate from medicine. Plants were sacred messengers. Roots, fruits, seeds, and leaves carried specific energies and frequencies—able to cool heat, tonify qi, calm the spirit, or build blood. Plants shaped the entire terrain of health and consciousness.

Today, quantum biology and nutrigenomics confirm this: food contains codes from the universe—encoded in its pigments, structures, and phytochemicals—that interact directly with your DNA. This is not metaphorical—it's biological. You are not just what you eat; you are what your body does with the information your food provides. Every bite tells your cells how to behave—to inflame or to calm, to grow or to repair, to store fat or burn fuel, or to degenerate or regenerate. And the most powerful, healing messages come in color.

EAT THE RAINBOW

Plants don't produce color for our entertainment. Their pigments are powerful compounds created to protect themselves from UV light, pathogens, and environmental stress. When we eat them, these same molecules activate cellular repair, fight inflammation, neutralize free radicals, and even support stem cell renewal. The deeper and more vibrant the color, the more antioxidants and healing phytochemicals the plant likely contains. This is why a beige, ultra-processed diet is a disease-promoting diet, whereas a diet filled with color is deeply therapeutic.

UNDERSTANDING ANTIOXIDANTS: THE BODY'S CELLULAR GUARDIANS

Antioxidants are compounds found in colorful plants that protect your cells from oxidative stress—the damaging effects of free radicals. Free radicals are unstable molecules generated by normal metabolism, pollution, stress, toxins, and even sunlight. When left unchecked, they damage DNA, accelerate aging, and increase the risk of chronic diseases.

Antioxidants work by donating electrons to stabilize free radicals, stopping the chain reaction of cellular damage. But they're not all the same—each antioxidant has a unique job, targets different systems, and works best under specific conditions. Let's explore the main types of antioxidants.

Lycopene, found in tomatoes (especially cooked), watermelon, red grapefruit, guava, and red bell peppers, is a powerful anti-inflammatory and anti-cancer compound. It protects the prostate, lungs, and cardiovascular system, and shields skin from UV damage.

Bioavailability tips: Heating tomatoes increases lycopene absorption by breaking down cell walls. Pair with a healthy fat (olive oil) to boost uptake.

Beta-carotene and **alpha-carotene** are precursors to vitamin A that are essential for your vision, immune health, and skin. They support reproductive health and epithelial tissues (gut lining, lungs), and can be found in carrots, sweet potatoes, pumpkins, mangoes, and cantaloupe. Bioavailability tips: Light steaming improves absorption. Pair with fat (ghee, avocado) for optimal conversion to vitamin A.

Lutein and **zeaxanthin**—found in spinach, kale, corn, egg yolks, yellow peppers, and marigold petals—essentially act like natural sunglasses for your eyes. They concentrate in the macula, where they absorb harmful blue light before it can damage delicate retinal tissue. This "filtering" not only protects your vision at the cellular level—it also sharpens contrast, reduces glare sensitivity, and makes bright light or night driving more comfortable. Lutein and zeaxanthin also support brain health and improve cognitive function.

Bioavailability tips: These are fat-soluble, so eat them with oil (like a kale salad with olive oil and lemon). Egg yolks boost absorption due to phospholipids.

Chlorophyll purifies blood, binds toxins, supports liver detoxification, and promotes alkalinity and cellular oxygenation. It can be found in all green leafy vegetables, chlorella, spirulina, parsley, and wheatgrass.

Bioavailability tips: It is best consumed raw or lightly steamed. Juicing greens or taking chlorophyll drops can deliver a concentrated dose.

Sulforaphane and **glucosinolates**—found in broccoli sprouts (richest source), kale, mustard greens, cabbage, and brussels sprouts—activate phase II liver detox enzymes, neutralize carcinogens, reduce inflammation, and protect DNA.

Bioavailability tips: Chop cruciferous veggies and let them sit for 10 minutes before cooking to activate enzymes. Light steaming preserves sulforaphane; avoid boiling.

Anthocyanins protect your brain, eyes, and blood vessels. They reduce oxidative stress and inflammation, promote neuronal regeneration and cognitive function, and support stem cell activation and longevity. Anthocyanins are found in blueberries, blackberries, purple sweet potatoes, red cabbage, black rice, and elderberries.

Bioavailability tips: These are best absorbed when paired with a healthy fat. Eat raw or lightly cooked; freezing doesn't destroy their potency.

Resveratrol and **pterostilbene** extend the lifespan in cells (linked to sirtuin activation), protect the brain and heart, and improve insulin sensitivity and mitochondrial health. They are found in red grapes (especially skins), blueberries, Japanese knotweed, and peanuts.

Bioavailability tips: Resveratrol has low oral bioavailability. It is best combined with fat and quercetin. Fermented grape products (like red wine in moderation) enhance absorption.

Quercetin is a natural antihistamine and anti-inflammatory. It supports lung health, immunity, and allergy relief, and enhances zinc transport into cells (important for viral defense). It is found in onions, apples (with skin), capers, parsley, and grapes.

Bioavailability tips: Combine with vitamin C to boost absorption. Cook onions gently to concentrate quercetin without destroying it.

A broad class of antioxidants that improve gut flora, blood sugar, and cognitive health, **polyphenols** reduce oxidative stress system-wide. They are found in green tea, dark chocolate, olives, extra virgin olive oil, blackberries, and coffee.

Bioavailability tips: They are best absorbed when taken with fiber-rich foods. Choose high-quality, minimally processed sources (e.g., ceremonial matcha, stone-pressed olive oil).

OTHER POWERFUL ANTIOXIDANTS

Vitamin C, the classic protector, is one of the most powerful water-soluble antioxidants. It protects blood and connective tissues, regenerates Vitamin E, supports collagen production, and strengthens immunity. Found in citrus, kiwi, bell peppers, camu, and acerola cherry, it quenches free radicals throughout the body.

Bioavailability tip: Pair with flavonoids (like quercetin) to boost absorption and synergy.

Vitamin E (tocopherols & tocotrienols) is the fat-soluble guardian of your cell membranes. While tocopherols are well known, tocotrienols (from annatto, palm fruit, and rice bran) are far more potent—up to 60x stronger in antioxidant capacity. Tocotrienols uniquely protect the nervous system, heart, and skin, and have remarkable anti-inflammatory and anti-cancer properties.

Bioavailability tip: The annatto plant provides the purest form of tocotrienols without tocopherol interference.

CoQ10 (ubiquinone & ubiquinol) is the mitochondrial defender. It is both an antioxidant and a vital player in energy (ATP) production inside the mitochondria. Levels decline with age, leaving the heart, brain, and muscles vulnerable to oxidative stress. CoQ10—especially the ubiquinol form—protects the cardiovascular system and supports vibrant energy.

Bioavailability tip: It is found in oily fish and organ meats, but supplementation is often essential.

Glutathione, the master antioxidant, is produced by your own cells—and it is the body's ultimate defense system. It neutralizes free radicals, recycles vitamins C and E, and drives liver detoxification. Chronic stress, toxins, alcohol, and aging deplete it quickly.

Bioavailability tip: Boost your glutathione naturally with sulfur-rich foods (garlic, onions, broccoli) or precursors like NAC and alpha-lipoic acid.

Alpha-Lipoic Acid (ALA), is the universal recycler and is unique because it works in both water and fat environments. It regenerates other antioxidants, improves blood sugar balance, and supports nerve health.

Bioavailability tip: ALA is found in spinach and organ meats but is best taken as a supplement.

Astaxanthin, the super carotenoid, is one of the most potent free radical quenchers ever discovered. Astaxanthin protects skin from UV damage, boosts endurance, and supports brain and eye health. Its unique structure allows it to span cell membranes, shielding both inside and outside layers.

Bioavailability tip: This deep-red antioxidant comes from microalgae, krill, and wild salmon.

Curcumin, the golden warrior, combines antioxidant power with profound anti-inflammatory effects. It protects the brain, heart, and joints, lowers oxidative stress, and enhances detoxification pathways.

Bioavailability tip: From turmeric, curcumin is best absorbed when combined with black pepper (piperine) and fat.

So, how can you maximize antioxidant intake in real life?

- Bless your food—your intention enhances assimilation.
- Eat at least three to five colors per meal.
- Lightly cook or combine with fat for better absorption (especially fat-soluble compounds).
- Rotate your colors weekly to activate different healing pathways.
- Add herbs and spices (like turmeric, rosemary, thyme)—they're small but potent antioxidant powerhouses.
- Juicing, fermenting, and blending can make certain compounds more bioavailable.
- Don't overcook—steam or roast gently instead of boiling or frying.

The deeper truth: Eating the rainbow isn't just about variety. It's about activating your innate cellular intelligence. Think of these pigments as keys unlocking different healing pathways inside you.

- Blue and purple support neurogenesis and emotional healing.
- Green strengthens your liver and blood.
- Red improves your circulation and vitality.
- Yellow and orange support digestion and immunity.
- White tones the lungs and gut.

Even more exciting, research now shows certain plant pigments can activate human stem cells, particularly deep blues and purples like those found in blueberries, purple sweet potatoes, and elderberry. This opens new doors in regenerative health and healthy aging.

RAINBOW MEDICINE CHECKLIST

RED

Key Antioxidants: lycopene, anthocyanins
Top Foods: tomatoes, strawberries, red cabbage, goji berries
Main Health Benefits: heart health, circulation, skin protection, inflammation reduction

ORANGE

Key Antioxidants: beta-carotene, alpha-carotene
Top Foods: carrots, sweet potatoes, pumpkin, mango
Main Health Benefits: vision, immunity, reproductive health

YELLOW

Key Antioxidants: lutein, zeaxanthin
Top Foods: corn, yellow peppers, squash, turmeric
Main Health Benefits: eye protection, brain function, blue light filtration

GREEN

Key Antioxidants: chlorophyll, sulforaphane
Top Foods: kale, spinach, broccoli, parsley, chlorella
Main Health Benefits: liver detox, hormone balance, blood building, alkalinity

BLUE

Key Antioxidants: anthocyanins, pterostilbene
Top Foods: blueberries, purple sweet potatoes, black rice
Main Health Benefits: brain and nervous system health, stem cell activation, anti-aging

PURPLE

Key Antioxidants: resveratrol, anthocyanins
Top Foods: grapes, eggplant, elderberries, purple cabbage
Main Health Benefits: longevity, cognitive protection, heart health, sirtuin activation. (Sirtuin activation means turning on a family of "longevity genes" that regulate cellular repair, metabolism, and inflammation. When activated—through certain nutrients, fasting, or stress-hormesis—sirtuins help protect DNA, improve mitochondrial function, and extend the health span of your cells.)

BLACK

Key Antioxidants: polyphenols, flavonoids
Top Foods: black garlic, black beans, black rice, plums
Main Health Benefits: blood sugar regulation, microbiome diversity, antioxidant resilience

WHITE

Key Antioxidants: quercetin, allicin, inulin
Top Foods: garlic, onions, cauliflower, mushrooms
Main Health Benefits: immunity, lung and gut health, antihistamine effect, microbiome support

TEN QUESTIONS TO ASK BEFORE YOU EAT

1. Is this food alive or processed?
2. Will this nourish or deplete my energy?
3. Is this real food or just an edible product?
4. How will I feel 30 minutes after eating this?
5. Is this choice supporting my goals or sabotaging them?
6. Am I truly hungry, or just bored, stressed, or triggered?
7. Was this food made with care—or with chemicals?
8. Would I feed this to someone I love?
9. Is there color, variety, and life on my plate?
10. Will this help me heal, or push me farther from balance?

Nature doesn't make junk food. Every plant is here with a purpose. Every color is a message from the Earth and the heavens, designed to feed not just your body—but your soul. Let food be your daily medicine, your spiritual nourishment, and your most loyal healer.

#7: LIVE WITH RHYTHM

You are not a machine. You are a rhythmic, pulsing, dynamic organism—a living system meant to flow with the natural cycles of the Earth.

The Vikings lived with rhythm. They rose with the sun. They ate what the land gave them in each season. They rested deeply in winter and moved powerfully in summer. They lived in tune with the world around them.

Modern life, by contrast, is chaotic, fast, artificial, and disconnected. We work through the night, eat under fluorescent lights, stare at blue screens before bed, and ignore our body's cries for stillness and renewal. When we lose rhythm, we lose health. When we restore rhythm, we restore harmony.

Your body runs on circadian rhythms, seasonal cycles, and biological timing. Every organ, hormone, and brain chemical is influenced by light, darkness, temperature, food, and sleep.

When you honor these rhythms, your systems run smoothly:

- ✓ Your digestion works better.
- ✓ Your hormones stay balanced.
- ✓ Your energy stabilizes.
- ✓ Your sleep becomes restorative.
- ✓ Your mood lifts.
- ✓ Your immune system strengthens.

When you push against your natural rhythm, your body pushes back with:

- ✗ Fatigue
- ✗ Anxiety or irritability
- ✗ Cravings and blood sugar crashes
- ✗ Sleep disturbances
- ✗ Hormonal imbalances
- ✗ Weakened immunity and inflammation

Rhythm isn't a luxury—it's a biological necessity.

CIRCADIAN RHYTHMS

Circadian rhythms are your body's internal 24-hour biological clocks that regulate everything from sleep-wake cycles to hormone release, digestion, metabolism, body temperature, and cellular repair. These rhythms are synchronized by a master clock in the brain called the suprachiasmatic nucleus (SCN), located in the hypothalamus. The SCN receives direct input from the retina, which detects light and darkness. This is why light is the strongest environmental cue (zeitgeber) for circadian regulation. But the SCN is not the only clock: Nearly every organ, tissue, and individual cell in your body has its own circadian clock, known as peripheral clocks. These are synchronized by the master clock—but they can also be influenced by other cues like food timing, temperature, and activity.

Circadian rhythms control the timing of many vital processes:

Brain Function and **Sleep**—Melatonin (the sleep hormone) rises at night when it's dark, helping you fall asleep. Cortisol (your stress/alertness hormone) rises in the early morning to help you wake up. Disruption leads to poor memory, brain fog, anxiety, and depression.

Immune System—Immune cell activity follows a circadian pattern. At night, the body shifts toward repair and inflammation control. Disruption leads to chronic inflammation, impaired healing, and weakened defenses.

Metabolism and **Digestion**—Insulin sensitivity and digestive enzyme release are highest earlier in the day. Eating late at night leads to higher blood sugar, increased fat storage, and insulin resistance over time.

Cellular Repair and **Detox**—Autophagy (cell cleanup), DNA repair, and liver detoxification peak at night during deep sleep. Disruption impairs cellular renewal, increasing the risks for cancer, aging, and chronic disease.

WHAT HAPPENS WHEN YOU WORK AT NIGHT OR STAY UP LATE?

Night shift work or late-night living creates circadian misalignment—a mismatch between your body's internal clock and the external world.

Scientific research has found:

- Higher rates of obesity, diabetes, cardiovascular disease, and cancer among night shift workers
- Increased depression, anxiety, and sleep disorders
- Disruption of melatonin production, which is also a potent antioxidant and cancer protector
- Impaired glucose tolerance and metabolism, leading to weight gain even with the same calorie intake

A 2017 review published in *The Lancet Diabetes & Endocrinology* stated that chronic circadian disruption is an independent risk factor for metabolic disease—regardless of diet or exercise.

To support healthy circadian rhythms naturally:

- ✓ Wake up and get sunlight exposure within 30 minutes of rising. This resets the suprachiasmatic nucleus (SCN) in your brain and supports cortisol rhythm.
- ✓ Eat meals during daylight hours. Avoid late-night eating to support metabolic and digestive clocks.
- ✓ Dim lights after sunset. Avoid blue light (screens) before bed to allow melatonin to rise.
- ✓ Sleep in total darkness. Even small light exposure at night can disrupt melatonin.
- ✓ Follow regular sleep and wake times—even on weekends. Consistency helps all systems sync.

SEASONAL RHYTHMS

Seasonal rhythms are biological shifts that happen in your body in response to changes in light, temperature, food availability, and environmental cues throughout the year. These are encoded in your DNA—passed down from ancestors who had to adapt to seasonal scarcity, cold, heat, and abundance. Light exposure shifts sleep cycles, thus naturally changing the melatonin and cortisol levels in your body. Appetite and metabolism are affected seasonally as well: Cold increases calorie needs; heat suppresses hunger. Thyroid, adrenal, and reproductive hormones also naturally adapt to conserve or expend energy. Your body increases its overall immune surveillance in the fall/winter, whereas there's more regeneration in the spring/summer.

In Chinese medicine, each season corresponds with a different organ system and emotional energy:

Seasonal Rhythms				
Season	Element	Organ	Emotion	Focus
spring	wood	liver	anger	detox, movement, cleansing, renewal
summer	fire	heart	joy	expansion, social connection
late summer	earth	spleen	worry	grounding, digestion, harvest
fall	metal	lungs	grief	letting go, breath, immunity
winter	water	kidneys	fear	rest, repair, deep nourishment

This wisdom mirrors modern science, which acknowledges seasonal shifts in immunity, mood, hormones, and metabolism. For example, thyroid hormones peak in winter to keep the body warm and metabolism active. Vitamin D and serotonin levels drop in fall/winter, affecting mood and immune resilience. Testosterone and reproductive hormones shift with photoperiod (daylight length). And studies show people have different inflammatory markers, cortisol rhythms, and fat-burning efficiency depending on the time of year.

When you align with seasonal rhythms, you don't need to force healing. You simply create the conditions for your body to thrive:

- ✓ Hormones stabilize.
- ✓ Sleep improves.
- ✓ Mood balances.
- ✓ Digestion regulates.
- ✓ Immune system strengthens.
- ✓ You age slower and feel more connected to your body and the earth.

When you fight the seasons—like eating cold smoothies in the winter or staying up late in darkness—you disrupt hormonal rhythms, weaken immunity, and feel chronically depleted.

Remember, you are not separate from nature—you *are* nature. The same force that turns the tides, blooms the flowers, and sheds the leaves is beating inside your body. The earth shows you how to heal—if you just listen. Let your food, movement, sleep, and rituals evolve with the seasons. Let each season guide a different phase of your healing, and rediscover what it means to live in harmony with the earth—and with yourself. Below are some tips on how to align with each season for optimal health.

WINTER (January–March): Rest and Restore

Theme: Slow down, nourish deeply, and reset your nervous system.

Rituals & Practices:
- » Sip bone broth or mushroom teas (reishi, chaga, lion's mane) daily or weekly.
- » Create candlelight evenings and aim for earlier sleep.
- » Enjoy warming adaptogens like ashwagandha, cinnamon, and ginger—perfect with journaling.
- » Dedicate one evening or morning a week to no technology and quiet reflection.
- » Move gently—yoga, stretching, or restorative walks.
- » Eat warming, mineral-rich foods and supplement with magnesium.
- » Reduce screen time—especially no screens 2 hours before bed.

Seasonal Focus: More rest, less stimulation, and steady nourishment for body and mind

SPRING (April–June): Awaken and Detox

Theme: Cleanse the liver, clear out the old, and step into renewal.

Rituals & Practices:
- » Support liver and gallbladder health with the Liver and Gallbladder Flush (see page 91).
- » Sip dandelion or nettle infusions to nourish and detox.

- » Begin a parasite cleanse with garlic, clove, and wormwood.
- » Declutter your space to refresh your mind and energy.
- » Stimulate detox with daily dry brushing or sauna sessions.
- » Eat greens with every meal and hydrate with birch sap or chlorophyll water.
- » Keep the colon moving with fiber, magnesium, and daily movement.
- » Use a letting-go ritual—write down what no longer serves you, then safely burn it.

Seasonal Focus: Lighten the body and mind—make space for growth and new energy.

SUMMER (July–September): Energize and Expand

Theme: Vitality, strength, mental clarity, and joy

Rituals & Practices:
- » Embrace wild swimming or refreshing cold plunges.
- » Get early morning sunlight for vitamin D and circadian rhythm support.
- » Ferment your own foods—sauerkraut, yogurt, or pickles.
- » Move outdoors—barefoot hiking, beach walks, or strength training in nature.
- » Favor light, fresh meals: salads, seasonal berries, and grilled fish or plant proteins.
- » Eat outside daily and breathe deeply with the sunrise.
- » Play, laugh, and create joy—let your nervous system recharge.
- » Take omega-3s daily to sharpen focus and protect your brain.

- » Connect with the earth through a weekly grounding ritual—ocean dip, forest time, or barefoot walk.

Seasonal Focus: Expand your energy, feed your joy, and soak in the season's abundance.

FALL (October–December): Ground and Prepare

Theme: Immune building, gut healing, and ancestral honoring

Rituals & Practices:
- » Nourish with bone broth and medicinal mushrooms (reishi, chaga, shiitake).
- » Create a seasonal altar with herbs, stones, and minerals that inspire you.
- » Focus on fall ferments—root vegetables, garlic, and sauerkraut for gut health.
- » Practice daily breath work or prayer to center the mind and body.
- » Honor your ancestors through seasonal foods, gatherings, or ritual offerings.
- » Include immune tonics like elderberry syrup, chaga tea, and zinc-rich foods.
- » Sip warm herbal teas and enjoy grounding meals like roasted root vegetables.
- » Take slow walks in nature to align with the season's slower rhythm.
- » Begin establishing winter habits—earlier evenings, deeper rest, and more stillness.

Seasonal Focus: Strengthen your foundation so winter's rest becomes a true restoration.

LIFESTYLE RHYTHM

The human body thrives on oscillation—periods of activity followed by periods of rest. This is known in science as the ultradian rhythm (every 90–120 minutes), and it scales upward: We need rest every day, every week, every month, and every year to prevent burnout, reset our hormones, and allow true regeneration. Without pause, stress hormones, such as cortisol and adrenaline, remain chronically elevated, leading to adrenal fatigue, hormonal imbalances, leaky gut and inflammation, anxiety, sleep issues, and emotional burnout. The antidote? Sacred rest, nature, and ritualized recovery. Below are the lifestyle rhythm practices to weave into your life.

Weekly Digital Detox (one day/week): Modern devices hijack your brain's dopamine system, fragment your focus, and overstimulate your nervous system. A weekly digital detox resets your brain chemistry and restores your ability to feel present. Try one day per week with no social media, emails, or screens. Replace screen time with books, music, journaling, cooking, nature, and face-to-face connections. Benefits include improved mental clarity, mood regulation, less anxiety, and better sleep.

Sabbath or **Sacred Pause Day**: All ancient cultures practiced a form of weekly rest—a Sabbath—not just for spiritual purposes but to reconnect to the soul, family, and inner stillness. Set aside one day each week for no productivity. Focus on nourishment—prayer, meditation, nature walks, long meals, and reflection. Benefits include deep parasympathetic healing, improved intuition, and spiritual alignment.

Weekly Nature Rhythm (at least 2 hrs./week): Nature is not just peaceful, it's biologically healing. Trees release phytoncides that enhance Natural Killer cell activity, reduce blood pressure, and reset brain waves into calm focus. Try forest bathing, beach walks, hikes, barefoot grounding, and gardening. Leave your phone behind, and just breathe and listen. Benefits include a reset for your nervous system, an immune boost, emotional regulation, and time for creativity.

Monthly Body Cleanse (new moon or full moon): Your body benefits from a mini-reset each month—especially around the new moon (cleansing energy) or the full moon (release). This supports your lymph, liver, and hormones. Try one to two days of light eating: broths, herbal teas, wild greens, and fruit. Include castor oil packs, dry brushing, sauna, or bitters. Benefits include a digestive reset, hormone recalibration, and enhanced intuition and clarity.

Annual Retreat or **Sacred Journey**: You need a pattern interrupt every year—a time away from the noise of daily life to reflect, realign, and restore your vision. This could be a healing retreat, a spiritual journey, or a solo trip into nature. Plan one retreat or sacred trip per year—even if it's just a weekend—to journal, fast, hike, or participate in a structured detox or emotional healing process. Benefits include a recalibrated purpose, the cleansing of emotional baggage, and renewed vitality and focus.

\	The Lifestyle Rhythm Map	
Frequency	Practice	Purpose
daily	sleep, hydration, meal timing	restore energy, reset metabolism, maintain rhythm
weekly	digital detox, sabbath	reconnect to self, nervous system reset
weekly	nature time	grounding, immune system, brain clarity
monthly	body cleanse	support liver, hormones, emotional detox
yearly	retreat or journey	soul alignment, life vision, deep repair

REFLECTION:
RHYTHM IS THE LANGUAGE OF HEALTH

In a world of endless health trends, biohacking, and miracle supplements, it's easy to forget the truth that has guided human vitality for millennia: The healthiest life is not built by intensity and force, but by rhythm.

Your body is not random. It is rhythmic. It follows patterns shaped by light and dark, sun and moon, tides and seasons. Your biology is still wired for Earth's original clock. When you align with that clock—sleeping with the sun and waking with the light; eating with the day and resting your digestion at night; cleansing in spring, nourishing in winter, letting go in the fall; pausing weekly, retreating yearly, and touching nature as often as you breathe—you unlock your body's innate intelligence. Your inflammation is reduced without pills. You balance hormones without forcing. You age slowly, beautifully, and powerfully. This is the rhythm of your ancestors. The rhythm of your organs. The rhythm of the earth. And it's the rhythm that brings you home to yourself. Let this be your new health strategy—not another fad or extreme, but a return to what is real, ancestral, and already inside of you. Live with rhythm, and your body will remember how to heal.

#8: LIVE WITH PURPOSE, INTENTION, AND ANCESTRAL MEANING

The Vikings didn't just live—they lived with conviction. Every harvest, every battle, every song, every prayer—they all served a purpose. They moved with intention. They ate to prepare. They trained for the future. They endured harsh winters because they believed something greater was waiting.

In our world of endless convenience and distraction, many have lost that sense of purpose. But without it, we drift. We decay. Purpose fades—and so does the life force. This is what modern retirement often looks like. Purpose is the fire that keeps your soul and body alive. Purpose is not optional. It's oxygen.

HOW PURPOSE KEPT ONE WARRIOR ALIVE

In the harsh winter of 986 AD, on the icy coast of Greenland, a Viking settler named Thorkell Leifsson—a lesser-known cousin of Leif Erikson—faced what should have been a death sentence. During a hunting expedition with his clan, he fell into a glacial crevasse and shattered his lower back. Paralyzed from the waist down, he was dragged home on a makeshift sled, unable to walk, fight, or provide—essentially useless by Viking standards. In Viking culture, strength and utility were sacred. To lose function of your body was often seen as a reason to accept death or be left behind. But Thorkell refused.

He didn't fight to survive for himself. He fought because he believed his true purpose was not to conquer land or swing an axe—it was to pass on wisdom and ensure the survival of their people through stories and skill. So Thorkell began mentoring the young. He taught boys how to read the sky, map the currents, and identify medicinal herbs. He trained them to carve tools with precision. He relayed tales of the gods but always with a lesson beneath: "Strength is not just muscle. It's knowing what must be done when your body cannot help you."

Against all odds, Thorkell lived another sixteen winters—longer than many warriors in his clan. His mind remained sharp, his spirit stronger than ever, and his teachings became the foundation of Greenland's next generation of explorers. When he died, they didn't bury him as a broken man. They carved into his stone: "He was our compass."

Modern science now confirms what Thorkell embodied: Having a strong sense of purpose can lower cortisol, boost immunity, reduce inflammation, and even extend lifespan. Thorkell's body may have broken, but his purpose kept him alive—and made him unforgettable.

Researchers studying the Blue Zones (regions where people live the longest, healthiest lives) found that the number-one longevity factor wasn't diet, exercise, or even genetics. It was purpose. Studies from those Blue Zones—and Harvard research alike—show that people with clear purpose:

- Recover faster from illness
- Live longer after retirement or trauma
- Are less likely to develop depression or dementia
- Are more resilient after loss
- Have lower rates of heart disease, dementia, and depression
- Wake up with energy, curiosity, and connection

The nervous system listens when you have a reason to keep going. Purpose literally becomes your medicine. In Okinawa, Japan—one of the longest-living cultures in the world—they have a word: *ikigai*. It means "a reason to get up in the morning."

One study from the *Journal of Psychological Science* found that people with a strong purpose lived longer even if they weren't physically healthy.

When you have purpose, your brain produces dopamine and serotonin. Your immune system activates healing pathways. Your stress hormones balance. Your heart rhythm stabilizes. Your cells receive the message: "Stay alive. You are needed."

Pair your purpose with daily intention and gratitude, and you create a field of healing around your life: Intention organizes your day around meaning. Gratitude programs your nervous system to feel safe. Purpose gives you a reason to keep going.

DAILY RITUALS TO ANCHOR YOUR PURPOSE

- Start your day with a mantra or prayer: "Today I serve my purpose with strength and grace."
- Reflect each week: "What did I do that mattered?"
- Practice a three-minute gratitude ritual at bedtime.
- Tell your story—Vikings passed down wisdom through words.
- Ask yourself often: "What do I stand for? What legacy do I want to leave?"

INSPIRATION: THE SONG THAT KEPT US ALIVE

I want to share a true story from my own life—a story of resilience, identity, and the unshakable power of purpose. It is a piece of my past and a reminder that no matter how dark the world may seem, your why will always light the way.

There are memories that never leave you—not because they haunt you, but because they define you. I was a young girl growing up in Soviet-occupied Latvia. To the outside world, we were part of a mighty empire. But inside, we were quietly grieving. We had once been free, but then our freedom lived only in whispers. We weren't allowed to talk about the past. The borders were shut. Travel was forbidden. Our passports meant nothing. And inside the stores, the shelves were nearly always empty. If you wanted bread, milk, or even soap, you needed ration cards. I still remember the scratchy feel of those paper tickets in my pocket. But even more than scarcity, there was silence. A silence that tried to erase history, that tried to flatten our identity. And yet . . . something in us wouldn't let go. We didn't fight with guns or protests. We fought with songs.

We sang our folk melodies, passed down through generations, with tears in our eyes and fire in our hearts. We danced barefoot on grass, just as our ancestors had done. We spoke our language, even when it was discouraged, because it carried our soul. And through all of that, we remembered who we were. Purpose lived in every note we sang.

One night, my father—strong and proud—attended a friend's birthday. As the guests toasted and laughed softly in the candlelight, he lifted his glass and said what so many longed to say: "God bless Latvia." The next day, the KGB came for him. He was taken, questioned, held for three days—and we didn't know if he would come home. But he did.

He came back thinner, quieter . . . and stronger—because they couldn't take away what he believed. And we knew: If we still had our songs, our stories, and each other, we were not broken. Then, something miraculous happened. It was 1989. People across Latvia, Lithuania, and Estonia had had enough. One summer evening, millions of us stood together—men, women, and children. We formed a human chain that stretched over 600 kilometers, hand in hand, from the southern tip of Lithuania to the north of Estonia. We called it the Baltic Way.

There were no weapons. No violence. No speeches. Just people—standing side by side across countries . . . and singing.

Imagine that for a moment—an entire nation, united by hands and voices, humming with the frequency of purpose. It was our declaration: We are still here. We remember who we are. And we will be free again. And we were. The Soviet Union would collapse soon after. Latvia rose again, not because of force, but because of the unshakable power of human spirit, culture, and the belief that purpose is stronger than oppression.

You might never face an empire trying to silence you. But perhaps, like so many, you've been told to shrink, to give up, to forget who you are. Don't. Your purpose is your anchor. Your purpose is your compass. It's the song that keeps you alive when everything else feels lost. And if a small nation on the edge of the world could stand hand in hand against the darkness—and win—then so can you. Never forget your song. Never forget your why. Because when you live with purpose, you can survive anything. And more than that—you rise.

#9: THE NON-NEGOTIABLES—THE FIVE PILLARS YOU CAN'T THRIVE WITHOUT

Let's rebuild your life around what matters most. You can eat all the right foods and take all the supplements in the world, but unless you move, sleep, hydrate, connect, and feel joy—your body can't fully heal. These five lifestyle forces are nonnegotiable. They are what make the difference between simply surviving and fully thriving.

1. Movement—the Ancient Language of Health: The human body was designed to move—every single day, not to sit in front of screens all day long. Even the purest spring becomes stagnant if it doesn't flow. And your body, made of over 70 percent water, is no different. Movement boosts brain function, increases insulin sensitivity, improves circulation, and stimulates your lymphatic and detox systems.

Some studies even show that exercise is a stronger predictor of longevity than diet or genetics. A 2018 study in *JAMA Network* showed that high cardiorespiratory fitness reduced mortality risk more than quitting smoking. Movement enhances brain-derived neurotrophic factor (BDNF)—a compound that protects your brain and boosts mood and focus. And research also shows that rebounding, walking, and lifting weights stimulate mitochondrial renewal and fat-burning.

Best exercises by goal or body type:

- Low energy? Bodyweight strength, zone 2 cardio, sauna and stretch
- Stressed or inflamed? Walk, rebound, breath-led yoga

- Strong and stable? Strength training 2–3x/week, hikes, kettlebells
- Sluggish lymph? Rebounding, fascia rolling, dry brushing, and gentle bouncing

2. Hydrate to Radiate: Your cells are water-based systems. Every metabolic process—detox, digestion, cellular energy, hormone transport, brain communication—requires water. But not just any water—structured, mineral-rich, living water. Stagnant, chlorinated tap water can't bring the same vitality as spring water, herbal infusions, or energized hydration. How much water? Well, the general guideline is half your body weight in ounces (e.g., 150 lbs. = 75 oz./day). But that figure needs to increase with heat, sweat, sauna, or caffeine.

Other tips:

- Always add a pinch of unrefined sea salt, trace minerals, or chlorophyll to your water. Without minerals, hydration fails to penetrate the cells.
- Drink between meals, not during, to preserve stomach acid and not dilute digestive enzymes.
- Herbal infusions (like nettle, peppermint, or ginger) count as cellular hydration.
- A good morning ritual: warm lemon water with air-dried sea salt plus bentonite clay or minerals to re-mineralize and cleanse

3. Sleep—Where the Body Truly Heals: You can't out-supplement or out-hustle poor sleep. Sleep is your body's deepest healing state. It is when your body repairs, regenerates, balances hormones, and processes emotion. Your hormones reset, growth hormone is produced, melatonin (your master antioxidant) surges, and brain detox pathways open (glymphatic system). Whereas poor sleep is linked to weight gain, dementia, depression, and hormone disruption.

There are four stages of sleep:

- » Stage 1 (light sleep)—transition to sleep
- » Stage 2—body temp drops, heart rate slows
- » Stage 3 (deep/NREM)—physical repair of muscles, bones, and tissues; immune strengthening
- » Stage 4 (REM)—brain repair, sorting memories, emotions, and neural patterns; dreaming, emotional healing

Sleep cycles last about 90 minutes, and you want four to five full cycles per night (7–9 hrs. total). Optimize sleep by:

- ✓ No screens 90 minutes before bed
- ✓ Magnesium, reishi, lemon balm, or chamomile tea
- ✓ Sleep in complete darkness (blackout curtains).
- ✓ Cool room, grounding sheets, sleep mask
- ✓ Dim lights after sunset (candlelight, red bulbs).
- ✓ Go to bed before 10:30 p.m. for full hormonal reset.

4. Connection—the Number-One Longevity Factor: In every Blue Zone, from Sardinia to Okinawa, there's one consistent thread—people are deeply connected to community, purpose, and laughter.

One Harvard study followed people for seventy-five years and found the strongest predictor of longevity was quality relationships. They lived in tight-knit communities, they gathered often, they laughed daily, and they felt seen, heard, and valued.

Even one good relationship can shift your entire stress physiology. Human beings are wired for connection. Isolation = inflammation. Connection = regeneration.

Some Viking-inspired connection rituals include:

- Joining or building a tribe
- Weekly meals with family and loved ones
- Storytelling and singing
- Nature walks with others
- Group saunas or cold plunges
- Circle rituals or seasonal gatherings

5. Joy—the Highest Frequency: You weren't born to just survive. You were born to feel joy—not the surface kind, but the soul-level joy that arises from truth, alignment, nature, laughter, and love. According to spiritual teachers and consciousness researchers, joy vibrates even higher than love, second only to enlightenment.

Joy is healing, magnetic, and contagious. It rewires your brain, strengthens your heart, and opens you to higher purpose. How to tap into joy:

- Dance, sing, move with freedom; let your inner child play.
- Spend time with children or animals and only with people who uplift your spirit.
- Create something—art, food, music.
- Laugh—even at yourself.
- Be in awe—stargaze, watch the ocean, touch a tree, spend time in nature.
- Practice daily gratitude—even for the hard days.

BEGINNING YOUR JOURNEY

You now hold the blueprint to a life of energy, clarity, and resilience. These nine Viking-inspired principles are not trends. They are timeless truths—rooted in ancestral wisdom, confirmed by modern science, and designed for today's toxic world.

You don't need to be perfect. You just need to begin. Choose one principle to start with. Feel it shift your energy. Then add another. Let it become a lifestyle. Let it become your new normal. Your body remembers how to heal. Your spirit remembers how to thrive. Now, so do you. You are the healer and the warrior. This is the Viking way.

DETOX LIKE A VIKING

*The body becomes the battlefield when toxins rule.
Cleanse it, and you reclaim your sovereignty.*

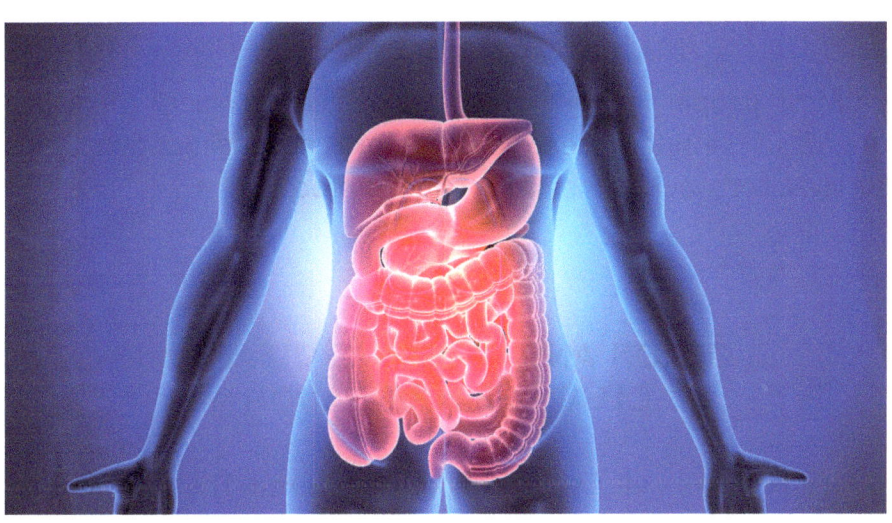

The Vikings didn't do juice cleanses. They didn't buy detox teas from influencers. They didn't need to. They lived in a world where the air was clean, the water was pure, the food was wild, and healing brews were made from wild herbs and fungi. Today's chemically saturated world, however, requires twenty-first-century Vikings to learn how to detox—proactively, consistently, and intelligently.

Why detox? Because toxins are silently disrupting your:

- ✓ Hormones
- ✓ Gut health
- ✓ Liver function
- ✓ Brain performance
- ✓ Immune system
- ✓ Fertility
- ✓ Mitochondria (your energy powerhouses)
- ✓ And your mood, clarity, and even spiritual awareness

Most people feel like they're "just getting older." In reality, they're just getting more toxic. So, detox is no longer optional—it's survival. Let's look at the Viking detox protocols.

COLON AND INTESTINAL CLEANSE: CLEAR THE FOUNDATION

No detox works well if your exit path is blocked. The colon is your body's waste chute—the final channel of elimination for toxins and waste. When it's clogged, inflamed, or sluggish, toxic debris builds up and gets reabsorbed into the bloodstream, taxing your liver, kidneys, lymph, and brain.

Your colon is also home to more than 70 percent of your immune system via the gut lining and is lined with trillions of microbes—your microbiome. It is responsible for the last stages of

nutrient absorption and is also key to hormone balance. Yes, your gut recycles estrogen!
A sluggish colon can lead to:

- Fatigue and brain fog
- Gas, bloating, constipation
- Skin breakouts and body odor
- Food sensitivities
- Mood issues and anxiety (via the gut-brain axis)
- Chronic inflammation

You *must* start with the colon before any deep detox—otherwise, you're just stirring up toxins with no exit. A clogged or inflamed colon not only slows elimination—it recirculates waste into the bloodstream, overburdens the liver, and weakens the immune system. That's why restoring gut integrity is the first step in healing.

WHAT DAMAGES THE GUT LINING (LEAKY GUT TRIGGERS)

- ✓ Processed foods and additives (like carrageenan, MSG, preservatives)
- ✓ Gluten and dairy (especially conventional forms)
- ✓ Refined sugar and alcohol
- ✓ Frequent antibiotic use or NSAIDs
- ✓ Chronic stress (elevates cortisol, weakens gut barrier)
- ✓ Lack of fiber and fermented foods
- ✓ Dehydration and irregular elimination

HOW TO DO THIS COLON CLEANSE

Over the course of three to five days, you're not using all of the ingredients at once, but rather combining a few based on your needs. The goal is to gently clear old waste, soothe inflammation, and prepare your body for deeper detox.

You can structure your daily colon cleanse like this (choose two to three daily):

- » Magnesium citrate or oxide—Take at night to encourage bowel movements (start with 400 mg and adjust as needed).
- » Psyllium husk or ground flaxseed—Take 1 tbsp. in water or juice in the morning or afternoon to bulk and sweep the intestines.
- » Aloe vera juice—Drink 1–2 oz. in water 1–2x daily to calm inflammation and support gut lining repair.
- » Triphala—Take one or two capsules or ½ tsp. powder at night for a gentle toning effect.

Optional additions (add one or two as needed):

- » Slippery elm or marshmallow root tea—Soothing for irritated bowels, 1–2x/day.
- » Activated charcoal or bentonite clay—Use away from food and supplements, 1–2x/day to bind released toxins.
- » Castor oil packs—Apply over the abdomen (or liver area) for 30–60 minutes, three or four times during the cleanse.
- » Enemas—Use herbal or warm filtered water enemas every other day to clear the lower bowel (if you feel sluggish or constipated).

» Colonics—Consider one or two professional colon hydrotherapy sessions during this 3–5-day window for a full flush.

TIPS FOR SUCCESS

Drink plenty of filtered water with minerals (like a pinch of sea salt) throughout the day. Eat light: focus on soups, broths, fruits, lightly steamed veggies, and easy-to-digest foods during the cleanse. Avoid heavy proteins, processed foods, dairy, gluten, and sugar while cleansing. Pay attention to how you feel—if anything feels too intense, pause and support your body with hydration, rest, and gentle movement. Avoid magnesium or psyllium if you have chronic loose stools or IBD; use soothing herbs instead.

How frequently should you cleanse your colon? Every one to three months or at the start of a seasonal or liver cleanse. If you've never done one, consider a full five-to-seven-day program to reset your gut. And be sure to do a colon cleanse before any liver flush or parasite cleanse.

CLEANSE DIET SUGGESTIONS

During any deep detox—especially colon, liver, or parasite cleansing—it's important to eat in a way that reduces digestive burden and supports elimination. This is not meant to be your forever diet, but rather a gentle, cleansing protocol for five to seven days while your body is working hard to flush out toxins.

Eat warm broths, soups, lightly cooked greens, and steamed, blended, or pureed vegetables. Drink gentle herbal teas like peppermint (for digestion), ginger (for circulation), senna (for bowel movement), and chamomile (for calming the nervous system). Avoid heavy meats, dairy, processed grains, caffeine, sugar, and alcohol.

POST-CLEANSE

Once you've cleared the colon and removed irritating triggers, it's time to rebuild and repair the gut lining. This phase is essential for restoring long-term digestive health, reducing inflammation, and preventing toxins from re-entering the bloodstream.

Support gut lining repair by doing as much of this as you can consistently for at least two to four weeks, or longer if you've had long-term gut issues. Even adding just a few of these daily can make a powerful difference over time:

- Aloe vera juice (inner fillet)—soothes inflammation and promotes tissue healing
- L-glutamine powder—the number-one fuel source for gut lining cells (enterocytes)
- Marshmallow, licorice root, slippery elm—herbal demulcents that coat and protect
- Probiotics or fermented foods restore microbiome balance and immunity.
- Bone broth or collagen—rich in glycine, proline, and healing amino acids
- Zinc carnosine, quercetin, and omega-3s reduce permeability, calm inflammation, and rebuild integrity.

DR. LAURA CAPINA

LIVER AND GALLBLADDER FLUSH—PURIFY YOUR FILTER AND BILE

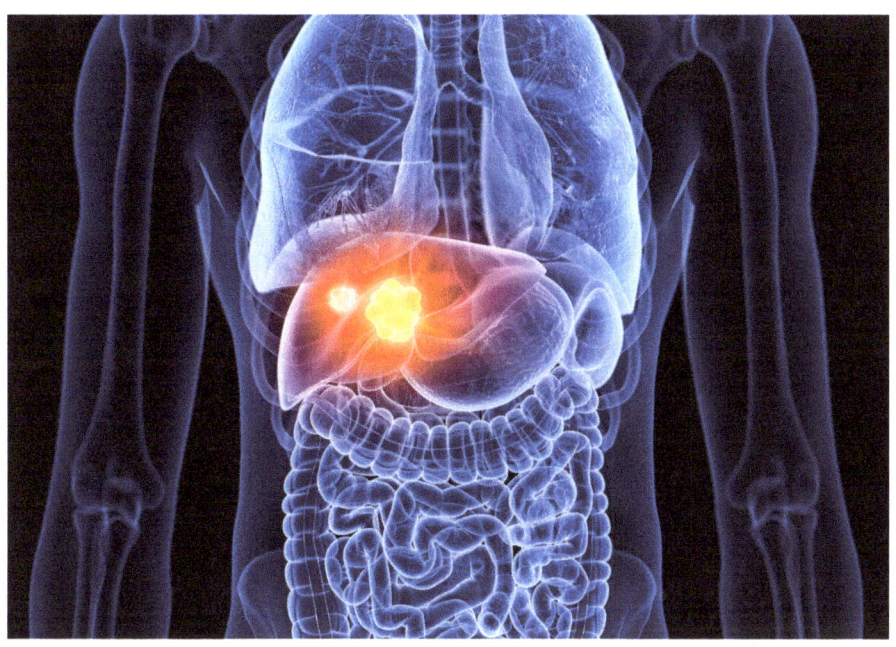

Once your colon is clear, the next priority is the liver and gallbladder—your body's central detox command center. The liver performs over 500 vital functions, including filtering your blood, neutralizing toxins, breaking down hormones, metabolizing fats, and producing bile, which is essential for digestion and detoxification.

When the liver is sluggish or congested, it cannot keep up with the daily onslaught of chemicals, stress hormones, environmental toxins, and inflammatory byproducts. As a result, waste begins to back up into the bloodstream, affecting every organ system—including your skin, brain, joints, and immune system.

A congested liver contributes to:

- ✓ Fatigue and brain fog
- ✓ Hormonal imbalances
- ✓ Skin breakouts and allergies
- ✓ Poor digestion, bloating, and constipation
- ✓ Blood sugar and cholesterol issues
- ✓ Stiff joints and blurred vision
- ✓ Irritability, frustration, and stored emotional heat (In Chinese medicine, liver governs anger and flow.)

The gallbladder works closely with the liver to store and release bile, which breaks down fats and carries toxins out of the body. If bile is too thick or the liver is clogged, digestion falters and detox stalls. This is why a liver cleanse—especially one that includes bile activation and gallbladder flushing—is absolutely essential for restoring energy, mental clarity, hormonal balance, and whole-body resilience.

You can't be truly healthy without a clean liver and gallbladder—period. Below I provide you with one of the most effective and time-tested protocols to remove bile sludge, stones, and stagnant toxins from the liver and gallbladder. This flush isn't for the faint of heart—but it can be life-changing for digestion, skin clarity, hormone balance, energy, and emotional well-being. It opens the bile ducts and helps purge the buildup that keeps your liver sluggish. Many people report releasing dozens or even hundreds of green, yellow, or tan stones from their liver and gallbladder—most of which go completely undetected in medical scans. After the cleanse, you might notice clearer skin, better digestion and elimination, hormonal balance (especially estrogen dominance), more energy and mental clarity, and an emotional release (the liver stores anger and resentment).

THE PREP PHASE (5–6 DAYS)

Drink one liter of organic apple juice or malic acid powder in water daily. This softens liver stones and prepares bile ducts. Eat light—mostly fruits, veggies, broths, and no fried or heavy foods. Stay hydrated, and keep bowels moving. (Colon cleansing is recommended before and after.)

FLUSH DAY (DAY 6 OR 7)

1. Stop eating by 2 p.m.
2. At 6 p.m., drink a glass of water with Epsom salts (magnesium sulfate)—about 1 tbsp. in ¾ cup water.
3. At 8 p.m., repeat the same Epsom salts drink.
4. At 9:45 p.m., mix ½ cup olive oil with ¾ cup fresh grapefruit or lemon juice—shake well. This stimulates a strong bile release and flush.
5. At 10 p.m., drink the olive oil and citrus blend in one go, lie down immediately on your right side with knees tucked for 20-30 minutes. Stay still and rest.

NEXT MORNING (DAY 7 OR 8)

At 6 a.m. and 8 a.m., take two more Epsom salts drinks. By mid-morning or afternoon, you'll begin to pass bile sludge and stones—often visible in the toilet as greenish or tan pebbles floating in the bowl.

Are you curious why Epsom salts is used in liver and gallbladder cleansing? It works by relaxing the smooth muscles of the bile ducts, allowing them to dilate and open more easily. This makes it less likely for bile or small stones to get stuck during the flush. Magnesium acts as a natural calcium channel blocker, which helps reduce spasms and supports the smooth release of bile. It also draws water into the colon, creating a gentle laxative effect that aids in flushing toxins and preventing reabsorption after the cleanse.

Tips: Do a colon cleanse the day before and/or after to prevent toxins from being reabsorbed. Stay home the next day—you'll need bathroom access and rest. Caution: Don't do this flush while pregnant, breastfeeding, very weak, or without support if chronically ill. Many people benefit from doing several flushes (every three to four weeks) until no more stones are released. After that, one to two seasonal flushes per year is great maintenance.

HOW TO SUPPORT YOUR LIVER EVERY DAY

Once you've done a liver flush, your next mission is to keep your liver flowing and protected every day. The liver is a high-performance organ—processing everything from food and emotions to toxins and hormones—but it needs your help to stay clean and efficient. Here are simple ways to support your liver daily:

Start your day with warm water and lemon juice or apple cider vinegar to stimulate bile and wake up digestion. Add in a pinch of unrefined sea salt to support mineral balance and hydration.

Eat liver-loving foods. Beets thin bile, boost methylation, and support phase-two liver detox. Bitter greens (arugula, dandelion, mustard greens, endive) stimulate bile flow. Cruciferous vegetables (broccoli, cauliflower, Brussels sprouts) are rich in sulforaphane for detox. Turmeric and black pepper are anti-inflammatory and liver protective. Milk thistle regenerates liver cells and buffers oxidative stress. Artichokes boost bile and protect liver tissue. Lemons, garlic, radish, cilantro, and parsley all help clear liver burden.

Hydrate intentionally: Drink half your body weight in ounces of water daily. Include lemon, chlorophyll, or herbal liver teas (dandelion, ginger, peppermint, burdock). Avoid ice-cold drinks, which shock digestion.

Castor oil packs are one of the oldest and most effective ways to reduce liver stagnation, inflammation, and hormonal imbalance. They help improve blood flow, move lymph, reduce congestion, and stimulate detox pathways.

What you'll need: organic castor oil, a flannel cloth or old T-shirt strip (folded to a palm-sized square), a hot water bottle or heating pad, and an old towel or clothing, because castor oil can stain.

Soak the cloth in castor oil until fully saturated (but not dripping). Place the cloth over your upper right abdomen (over the liver). Cover with plastic wrap or an old towel. Apply heat (hot water bottle or heating pad). Lie down and relax for 30-60 minutes. Optional: Meditate, breathe deeply, or listen to calming music while resting. Afterward, clean the area with warm water and baking soda or lemon.

Tips: Repeat 3-4x/week, especially after liver flushes or during cleanses. This is also great over the uterus or intestines to reduce cramping and inflammation.

KIDNEY AND BLADDER CLEANSE: RESTORE YOUR INNER WATERS

As I always tell my patients: The kidneys are the body's master filters, and the bladder is the exit door. If your inner waters are stagnant, toxins stay trapped.

The kidneys are two bean-shaped organs located on either side of the spine, just below the ribs. Each day, they filter over fifty gallons of blood and produce about one and a half quarts of urine, removing waste, excess water, and toxins. But they do far more than just make urine.

The kidneys:

- ✓ Filter blood and remove metabolic waste (urea, uric acid, heavy metals)
- ✓ Regulate electrolytes (sodium, potassium, magnesium)
- ✓ Maintain acid-alkaline balance (pH)
- ✓ Control blood pressure via the renin-angiotensin system
- ✓ Support red blood cell production via erythropoietin

- ✓ Regulate vitamin D activation for calcium metabolism

The urinary bladder stores and excretes urine. If it's inflamed, stagnant, or holding on to old toxins, you may experience burning, cloudy urine, frequent urination, or low-grade infection-like symptoms.

WHAT DAMAGES KIDNEY HEALTH

- ✓ Dehydration
- ✓ Overuse of ibuprofen, NSAIDs, antacids
- ✓ Smoking and alcohol
- ✓ High-sodium diets
- ✓ Heavy metal buildup (mercury, cadmium)
- ✓ Chronic stress (reduces kidney qi in TCM)

When the kidneys or bladder are burdened:

- ✗ Detox becomes impaired.
- ✗ Inflammation rises systemically.
- ✗ Fluid retention and puffiness occur.
- ✗ Hormonal and bone imbalances emerge.
- ✗ Fatigue, brain fog, and pain may worsen.

CLEANSING THE KIDNEYS AND BLADDER (GENTLE FLUSH, 7–10 DAYS)

This gentle cleanse is designed to hydrate, flush, and support the kidneys and urinary tract, without requiring fasting or extreme detox protocols. You'll be using a combination of herbal teas, tinctures, and supportive nutrients that work together to reduce inflammation, clear toxins, and strengthen these vital elimination organs.

Choose four to six of the herbs listed below and either brew them as loose tea or in pre-made blends (available at health food stores or online), or take them as liquid tinctures or capsules (always choose organic and alcohol-free when possible). Another option is to blend fresh herbs like parsley, cranberry, or nettles into a daily smoothie with lemon, cucumber, and filtered water.

Key herbs:

Uva ursi—antimicrobial, bladder tonic
Couch grass root—soothes inflammation
Corn silk—mild diuretic, urinary soother
Horsetail—strengthens bladder walls, rich in silica
Cranberry (whole fruit or extract)—reduces bacteria adhesion
Dandelion leaf—potassium-sparing diuretic
Parsley—natural kidney flush support
Nettle leaf—mineral-rich and anti-inflammatory

Tips: Focus on light, water-rich meals: cucumbers, melons, celery, leafy greens, radishes. Avoid salty, acidic, or high-oxalate foods (spinach, almonds, chocolate) during the flush.

Limit caffeine, alcohol, meat, and heavy fats for seven to ten days.Optional: Add a watermelon fast or juice for one or two days. This is very hydrating and cleansing.

Take supportive supplements once or twice daily with food. Supportive supplements include **magnesium** to relax bladder muscles, **B6** and **potassium citrate** to prevent oxalate buildup (stones), and **vitamin C** (non-acidic forms), as a mildly antimicrobial and alkalizing agent.

Fluid-wise, drink kidney flush teas 2–3x/day. Aim to stay hydrated with at least half your body weight in ounces of clean water daily, adding lemon, chlorophyll, or unsweetened cranberry juice if desired.

POST-CLEANSE

Even after your cleanse, your kidneys and bladder deserve ongoing love: Stay hydrated—make water your number-one beverage. Sip nettle or parsley tea a few times a week. Add celery juice, cucumber, lemon water, and greens to your daily diet. Avoid excess protein and processed salt. Replenish minerals—magnesium, potassium, silica, trace minerals—and reduce long-term NSAID use; they burden the kidneys. Practice deep breathing and emotional release.

EMOTIONAL AND ENERGETIC VIEW (TRADITIONAL CHINESE MEDICINE)

In Chinese medicine, kidneys are the seat of vital essence (*Jing*)—your life force and longevity. Courage and willpower are considered to reside within the kidneys. Fear, insecurity, or depletion manifest when the kidneys are weak. The bladder, on the other hand, governs releasing what no longer serves—physically and emotionally. When you strengthen these organs, you're not just detoxing—you're restoring your foundation and longevity.

HEAVY METAL DETOX: ELIMINATE THE SILENT SABOTEURS

No cleanse is complete without addressing heavy metals—because they block healing on every level. You can't see them. You can't smell them. But they're silently hijacking your brain, hormones, and immune system.

Metals like mercury, lead, arsenic, cadmium, and aluminum accumulate slowly—over decades—in your:

- ✓ Brain and nervous system (contributing to brain fog, anxiety, memory loss, neurodegeneration)
- ✓ Liver and kidneys (burdening detox and filtration)
- ✓ Bones and thyroid (displacing calcium, zinc, and iodine)
- ✓ Immune system (triggering inflammation, autoimmunity, and fatigue)

These metals don't leave the body easily. They bind tightly to tissues and can cross the blood-brain barrier, creating chronic low-level toxicity that affects nearly every system in your body.

Heavy metals can:

- Disrupt mitochondria (your energy production)
- Mimic or block minerals like zinc, magnesium, and selenium
- Contribute to mood disorders, neurological decline, and ADHD
- Exacerbate autoimmune conditions and leaky gut
- Increase your toxic load and inflammation

WHERE THEY COME FROM

- Dental mercury fillings (amalgams)
- Seafood (especially tuna, swordfish, mackerel)
- Tap water (lead, arsenic, aluminum)
- Certain vaccines and pharmaceuticals (aluminum adjuvants)
- Beauty products, deodorants, and cosmetics (aluminum, lead)
- Air pollution, gasoline fumes, chemtrails
- Cookware, pipes, pesticides, paints, and industrial exposure

Even if you eat clean today, decades of exposure can still be stored in your body—especially in fat tissue and the brain.

DENTAL MERCURY FILLINGS: A HIDDEN TIME BOMB

Silver amalgam fillings are up to 50 percent mercury. Every time you chew, grind, or drink hot liquid, vaporized mercury is released into your bloodstream and brain. Mercury crosses the blood-brain barrier, where it binds to fat and nerve tissue, damaging mitochondria, memory, and mood.

If you're doing a heavy metal cleanse but still have mercury fillings, you may just be redistributing metals. That's why removal—when done safely—can be life-changing. But NEVER remove amalgam at a regular dental office. Always choose a biological dentist certified in SMART protocol (Safe Mercury Amalgam Removal Technique).

Before removal:

- Open the colon and liver.
- Use binders 24–48 hrs. before and after.
- Support kidneys with teas or minerals.
- Ensure adequate selenium, zinc, and magnesium.
- Consider IV vitamin C or glutathione.

During/after removal:

- Space out fillings (one every three to four weeks if needed).
- Continue binders daily for two to three months.
- Support detox with sweating, hydration, and rest.
- Replenish minerals aggressively (especially selenium and sulfur-rich foods).

HOW TO CLEANSE HEAVY METALS SAFELY

A heavy metal cleanse is not just a detox—it's a deep-level rebuild. Core detox agents:

Chlorella—binds mercury, cadmium, lead
Spirulina—supports cell repair and detox
Cilantro—mobilizes metals from deep tissues (always pair with binders)
Zeolite clay—powerful binder for aluminum, lead, and more
Fulvic acid—helps transport toxins out of cells
Bentonite clay—absorbs metals and toxins in the gut
Activated charcoal or **modified citrus pectin**—bind toxins in the intestines

Instructions (cycle for one to three months): Start with binders (2–3x/week) away from meals and supplements. Add chlorella and spirulina to green smoothies or detox shots. Blend fresh cilantro into juices, soups, or pestos. Use zeolite or fulvic acid drops as tolerated. Pair with infrared sauna, rebounding, or dry brushing to support lymphatic drainage.

HOW TO SUPPORT DETOX DAILY

- ✓ Drink mineral-rich water with lemon, sea salt, or trace minerals.
- ✓ Take a binder 1–3x/week (empty stomach, 1 hr. away from food/supplements).
- ✓ Greens, seaweed, or chlorophyll daily

- ✓ Eat sulfur-rich foods (garlic, onions, broccoli, eggs).
- ✓ Add parsley, dandelion, cilantro, beets regularly.
- ✓ Rotate in chlorella, spirulina, and zeolite to bind and mobilize.
- ✓ Keep colon and liver flowing (sweating, movement, magnesium, hydration).

- ✗ Caution: Detoxing metals too fast can stir up toxicity and overwhelm the body, leading to headaches, fatigue, mood swings, skin eruptions, and nausea or flu-like symptoms. Always start small. Always use binders. And always support the colon, liver, kidneys, and lymph.

PARASITE CLEANSE— ELIMINATE HIDDEN INTRUDERS

You're not alone in your body—unless you make sure of it. It's estimated that 60–80 percent of people carry parasites—some visible (worms), others microscopic (protozoa, flukes). They often go undetected for years, but the symptoms they cause can be life-altering.

We're exposed through:

- » Undercooked meat, sushi, pork, and contaminated water
- » Pets (especially cats and dogs), livestock, and insects
- » Traveling to tropical or rural regions
- » Poor hygiene or food handling
- » Soil, gardening, or barefoot walking

Most people don't realize they have them until they do a cleanse and feel dramatically better afterward.

SYMPTOMS OF PARASITE LOAD

Parasites often cause nonspecific symptoms that mimic other conditions, including:

- ✓ Bloating, gas, IBS
- ✓ Itchy skin, rashes, eczema
- ✓ Brain fog, fatigue, mood swings
- ✓ Teeth grinding, especially at night
- ✓ Nutrient deficiencies despite healthy eating
- ✓ Anxiety, irritability, or unexplained anger
- ✓ Cravings for sugar and carbs
- ✓ Trouble sleeping or waking at 3–4 a.m.

Some parasites release neurotoxins, steal nutrients, and disrupt your immune system—leading to food sensitivities, autoimmune symptoms, and chronic inflammation.

TOP PARASITE-FIGHTING TOOLS

These herbal powerhouses are most effective in combination formulas or tinctures.

- **Black walnut hull** kills adult parasites and cleanses the blood.

- **Wormwood** (Artemisia) is one of the strongest antiparasitic herbs.
- **Clove** targets eggs and larvae (crucial for breaking the cycle).
- **Mimosa pudica seed** is a sticky seed that grabs and binds parasites in the gut.
- **Diatomaceous earth** (food-grade) are sharp micro-particles that slice parasite biofilms.
- **Papaya seeds** are potent natural antiparasitics.
- **Pumpkin seeds** paralyze parasites, especially tapeworms.
- **Garlic** is an antimicrobial, antifungal, and antiparasitic.

HOW TO DO A PARASITE CLEANSE (BEGINNER-FRIENDLY PROTOCOL)

Preparation (Week 1)

- Open your detox pathways first! For the colon: magnesium, fiber, water. For the liver: bitters, broths, lemon water. For the kidneys: tea, hydration.
- Take binders—charcoal, clay, or pectin—away from food.

Parasite Attack (Weeks 2–4)

- Use a trusted herbal blend or tincture with black walnut, wormwood, or clove.
- Add Mimosa pudica, DE, pumpkin seeds, garlic, and papaya seeds.
- Take twice/day, ideally with meals.
- Continue binders (1–2 hrs. away from herbs).

Rest and Rebuild (Week 5)

- Take a 5 to 7-day break to support your liver and gut.
- Load up on minerals, probiotics, and gut-healing foods.

Timing tip: Parasites are most active around the full moon. That's when your melatonin (which suppresses them) naturally drops, and serotonin (which they feed on) goes up. This makes them more mobile and easier to target. The ideal window for a parasite cleanse is from the new moon to the full moon—about 10 to 14 days. Do two to three cycles like this to hit all the stages: eggs, larvae, and adults.

Caution: When parasites die, they release toxins, ammonia, and inflammation. This can cause headaches, skin eruptions, fatigue, nausea or dizziness, and mood swings. Always start slow. Always support elimination: Detox baths, liver teas, and binders are your friends. You don't want to stir the swamp—you want to drain it carefully.

HOW TO PREVENT REINFECTION

Wash hands and nails regularly (especially after gardening or handling pets). Deworm your pets regularly, and use diatomaceous earth around pet areas. Clean bedding weekly during cleansing, and do not walk barefoot in tropical soil or contaminated water. Wash fruits and vegetables thoroughly, and avoid sushi, undercooked pork, and street food while traveling.

Supportive antiparasitic foods include:

- ✓ Raw garlic

- ✓ Papaya with seeds
- ✓ Pumpkin seeds (raw, ¼ cup/day)
- ✓ Pineapple
- ✓ Pomegranate
- ✓ Cloves and cinnamon
- ✓ Ginger, turmeric
- ✓ Fermented foods (sauerkraut, kefir, kimchi)

EMERGING SCIENCE AND ANCIENT INSIGHT

Parasites don't cause every cancer—but many cancers won't heal until parasites are addressed. While mainstream medicine doesn't often talk about it, researchers and holistic doctors have long observed a correlation between parasite burden and cancer. And modern science is starting to catch up. For example, *schistosoma haematobium*, a water-borne parasite, is now linked to bladder cancer; *opisthorchis viverrini* (liver fluke) is linked to cholangio-carcinoma (bile duct cancer); and *clonorchis sinensis* is associated with liver and gallbladder cancer.

Research has shown that:

- ✓ Parasites release toxic metabolic waste, ammonia, and enzymes that create chronic inflammation, disrupt cell communication, damage DNA over time, and suppress the immune system's ability to detect abnormal (cancerous) cells.
- ✓ Parasites thrive in low-oxygen, acidic environments, just like cancer cells. They feed on nutrients and steal minerals, weakening the body's ability to repair and defend.

- ✓ Cancer patients often test positive for parasitic infections. Some patients with stubborn or recurring cancer only improve after aggressive parasite cleansing.
- ✓ Parasite cleansing helps improve immune function, reduce inflammation, and restore vitality. In ancient systems like Chinese medicine and Ayurveda, cleansing parasites is a standard part of cancer prevention and treatment.

OTHER CONNECTIONS BEING EXPLORED

Parasites can create or hide in protective biofilms—slimy coatings that also harbor fungi, bacteria, and even cancer cells. Breaking down biofilms is key to healing.

Tissue burrowing: Some parasites burrow deep into organs, creating lesions or cysts that are mistaken for tumors or may develop into precancerous tissue.

The bottom line is, while parasites aren't the sole cause of cancer, they may:

- ✓ Contribute to the terrain that allows cancer to develop
- ✓ Suppress the immune system, allowing abnormal cells to grow unchecked
- ✓ Interfere with detox and nutrient absorption, slowing healing
- ✓ Increase toxic burden, acidity, and inflammation

Cleansing parasites is a foundational tool in any long-term healing strategy. If you're not clearing parasites, you might be missing a core piece of the puzzle.

SPIKE PROTEIN AND SYNTHETIC TOXIN CLEANSE—DEFEND AGAINST MODERN BIOLOGICAL INTERFERENCE

Detox what your body was never designed to handle. Spike proteins and synthetic materials introduced via mRNA exposure, viral infections, environmental toxins, and even passive shedding have created a new class of toxic burden—one that's difficult to clear using standard detox approaches.

Foreign proteins and materials:

- Bind to ACE2 receptors, interfering with blood pressure, immune balance, and cellular entry
- Cross the blood-brain barrier, contributing to neurological issues like brain fog, anxiety, and fatigue
- Trigger immune dysregulation and chronic inflammation
- Disrupt mitochondrial function, lowering energy and cellular repair
- Damage the vascular system, potentially contributing to clotting, long-haul symptoms, and endothelial inflammation

We are living in a biologically engineered toxic era—our detox tools must evolve with it.

HOW TO DETOX SPIKE PROTEINS SAFELY

The key is to combine antioxidants and nutrients that block spike binding and support immune function, proteolytic enzymes that break down residual proteins, herbal antivirals that inhibit replication, repair tissue, and support mitochondria, and binders and detox practices to ensure proper elimination.

Core Nutrient-Based Cleanse Stack		
Supplement	Dose	Function
NAC (N-acetylcysteine)	600–1200 mg/day	glutathione precursor, detox antioxidant, lung support
quercetin	250–500 mg/day	zinc ionophore, anti-inflammatory, blocks viral entry
zinc	25–50 mg/day	essential immune cofactor
vitamin D3 & K2	2000–5000 IU/day	immune modulation, inflammation control
vitamin C	1000 mg twice/day	antioxidant, immune support, collagen protection
omega-3s (DHA/EPA)	1000–2000 mg/day	anti-inflammatory, cellular repair

Enzyme Support for Protein Breakdown

Enzyme	Dose	Function
*nattokinase	100–200 mg/day	breaks down spike protein fragments, fibrin, supports circulation
*bromelain	250–500 mg/day	proteolytic enzyme, reduces inflammation, supports digestion of proteins
curcumin (from turmeric)	500–1000 mg/day	anti-inflammatory, neuroprotective, liver support

Avoid nattokinase and bromelain if on blood thinners or if you have a bleeding disorder. Always consult a qualified practitioner.

HERBAL ANTIVIRALS AND IMMUNE MODULATORS

These herbs go beyond fighting viruses—they also block spike binding, reduce inflammation, protect mitochondria, and support immune balance.

> **Pine needle** (shikimic acid) is a Nordic/Viking remedy that counteracts spike activity. It is a respiratory and immune tonic.

Japanese knotweed (resveratrol) inhibits spike binding, protects the cardiovascular system, and is used for Lyme disease and other long-haul viral issues.

Andrographis is a powerful immune regulator. It reduces cytokine storms and supports the lungs, lymph, and inflammatory control.

Artemisinin, from sweet wormwood, is effective against viruses and parasites. It may inhibit clotting and block spike interactions.

Chaga is a Viking-era birch fungus that is high in betulinic acid. It is an immune modulator, aids DNA repair, and is a gut-lung axis healer.

Garlic is a broad-spectrum antiviral that breaks biofilms and improves immunity.

Chinese skullcap (Scutellaria baicalensis) is a flavonoid that reduces spike inflammation. It is neuroprotective, an antiviral, and liver-safe.

Cat's claw breaks biofilms, modulates immunity, and repairs damaged tissue.

Licorice root supports the adrenals, lungs, and gut lining. It inhibits viral replication and binding.

SUPPORTIVE PRACTICES: ESSENTIAL FOR DETOX SUCCESS

- Infrared sauna or sweating (3–5x/week)
- Cold plunges or contrast showers to reduce inflammation
- Deep sleep (no screens 1–2 hrs. before bed)
- Gentle movement: yoga, walking, rebounding
- Breath work and vagus nerve activation to calm inflammation
- Binders: charcoal, zeolite, or pectin (take away from food/supplements)
- Hydration: add lemon, chlorophyll, or minerals to water
- Liver support: dandelion, milk thistle, castor oil packs

HOW TO CLEANSE

A Four-Week Suggested Protocol	
Week	Focus
Week 1	Start NAC, zinc, vitamin D, omega-3s, and quercetin. Begin hydrating more and prepping liver and colon. Add sauna or dry brushing.
Week 2	Introduce enzymes (nattokinase/bromelain) slowly. Begin herbal stack (three to five core herbs). Add binders 2–3x/week.

Week 3	Continue herbal protocol. Increase movement and breath work. Monitor reactions—adjust as needed.
Week 4	Focus on restoration: glutathione-rich foods, probiotics, light eating, deep sleep, grounding in nature.

Repeat in cycles as needed based on symptoms or exposure.

We are living in unprecedented biological terrain. But your body—when properly supported—knows how to clear, restore, and regenerate. Clean the terrain. Support your systems. Reclaim your strength.

LYMPH AND SKIN DETOX—KEEP YOUR DRAINAGE AND GLOW FLOWING

If your drains are clogged, the house backs up. Your lymph and skin are your detox drains—keep them open, and you stay clean. Your lymphatic system is your body's internal river. It bathes every cell, removes metabolic waste, transports immune cells, and acts as your second circulatory system. Unlike your heart, the lymph system has no pump—it relies entirely on movement, hydration, and breath to keep flowing.

If lymph becomes stagnant, it can cause:

- ✓ Puffiness, swelling, or cellulite
- ✓ Brain fog and fatigue

- ✓ Acne, rashes, or skin flare-ups
- ✓ Weakened immune function
- ✓ Sluggish detox and chronic inflammation

THE SKIN: YOUR LARGEST ORGAN OF DETOX

Your skin is not just a barrier—it's a major channel of elimination. It excretes toxins through sweat glands and pores and reflects what's happening inside your body, especially if the liver or lymph is overloaded. When detox pathways are blocked, toxins push out through the skin, leading to acne, eczema, and rashes; dullness or discoloration; premature aging; and body odor.

In Chinese medicine, skin and lungs are intimately connected. Sweat is one of the fastest ways to clear heat and toxins.

HOW TO CLEANSE THE LYMPH AND SKIN (DURING DETOX OR SEASONALLY)

Dry brushing stimulates lymph flow, exfoliates skin, and boosts circulation. Be sure to use a natural bristle brush, and brush before showering (2–3 minutes total). Always brush toward the heart. Start at the feet → legs → abdomen → arms → chest.

Rebounding (mini trampoline) moves stagnant lymph, oxygenates tissue, and tones the core. This gentle bouncing—feet barely leave the mat—is best done before a sauna or shower for 5–15 minutes per day.

Body scrubs remove dead skin, stimulate lymph, and energize the skin. Use once or twice/week, especially during detox or seasonal transitions. Try combining ½ cup sea salt or sugar and 2–3 tbsp. coconut or olive oil. Add essential oils: rosemary, grapefruit, peppermint. Apply in circular motions toward the heart. Then, rinse with warm, finish with cold water.

Castor oil packs improve liver flow and lymphatic movement and, when used before menstruation, can help ease cramps. Avoid applying directly to the lower abdomen during active bleeding or during pregnancy.

Clay masks pull toxins from armpits, the face, and feet. They are great for the lymph nodes. Once or twice a week for detox cycles, try mixing bentonite clay with apple cider vinegar (ACV) or water. Apply to face, armpits, hands, and feet. Let dry 10–20 minutes, rinse and moisturize.

Contrast showers work because the cold constricts and the hot dilates—pumping lymph and skin detox.

Infrared or traditional saunas help you sweat out toxins, boost circulation, and clear pores. Partake 2–4x/week.

Hydration and minerals are important because the lymph needs fluid and electrolytes to move and flush.

EVERYDAY LYMPH AND SKIN SUPPORT

- Walk daily (especially outdoors with deep breathing).
- Avoid tight bras and/or clothing that restricts lymph flow.
- Drink warm lemon water and minerals in the morning.
- Choose natural, nontoxic skin care (no endocrine disruptors).
- Fast occasionally or do light meals to give your system a break.
- Don't suppress sweat—it's one of your best detox tools.

Your lymph and skin are gatekeepers and messengers. When they're clear, glowing, and flowing—you'll feel lighter, clearer, and more resilient. To detox deeply, you must support your body's drainage systems.

MOLD TOXICITY—THE HIDDEN SABOTEUR

Mold isn't just an unsightly problem—it's a living organism that can silently infiltrate your home, body, and health. The fungus thrives in damp, dark environments—feeding on organic materials like wood, drywall, carpet, and even paper—and is far more common than most people realize. It often hides behind walls, under flooring, in air conditioning units, under sinks, inside washing machines, in basements, attics, or anywhere water damage has occurred. Even "minor" leaks or humidity issues can set the stage for mold growth. Because it spreads through microscopic spores, you may not see it—but you can still be breathing it in daily.

While there are thousands of mold species, black mold (*Stachybotrys chartarum*) is the most notorious. It produces mycotoxins—poisonous compounds that can severely damage human health. When mold spores or mycotoxins enter the body—through inhalation, ingestion, or skin contact—they can overwhelm the immune system and disrupt multiple organ systems. Mycotoxins can penetrate cell membranes, impair mitochondrial function, and create chronic inflammation. This often leads to multi-system illness that is notoriously difficult to diagnose.

COMMON SYMPTOMS

- Persistent fatigue and brain fog
- Sinus congestion or chronic cough
- Migraines and light sensitivity
- Muscle weakness or joint pain
- Digestive disturbances
- Anxiety, depression, or mood swings
- Skin rashes or itching
- Unexplained weight gain or loss
- Hormonal imbalances
- Heightened sensitivity to chemicals or smells

For some, mold exposure can be life-altering. I had a patient who moved into a home with hidden water damage. Within months, her energy plummeted, her mind felt clouded, and every system in her body seemed to unravel. Even after moving out, her health never fully recovered—the mycotoxin burden had triggered a cascade of chronic illness that stayed with her for life.

THE MOST POWERFUL MOLD DETOX STRATEGIES

1. Remove the source: You can't heal if you're still being exposed. Professional remediation is critical. Simply cleaning the surface won't remove mycotoxins from porous materials. Sometimes, belongings must be discarded.

2. Support drainage pathways: Open up the liver, lymph, kidneys, and colon before aggressive detoxing. Hydration, gentle movement, and castor oil packs can help.

3. Bind the toxins: Certain binders "catch" mycotoxins in the gut so they can be excreted. These include activated charcoal, bentonite clay, chlorella, and specific prescription binders (under medical guidance).

4. Boost antioxidant defense: Mycotoxins create oxidative stress. Glutathione, NAC (N-acetyl cysteine), vitamin C, and alpha-lipoic acid are potent protectors.

5. Heal the mitochondria: Mold damages your cellular "batteries." CoQ10, PQQ, and omega-3 DHA can help restore energy production.

6. Sweat it out: Infrared saunas and exercise can help release toxins through the skin.

7. Rebuild the gut: Mold disrupts microbiome balance. Probiotics, prebiotics, and gut-healing nutrients (like L-glutamine and aloe vera) are essential for repair.

Mold detox is not a quick fix—it's a layered, patient process. But with the right strategy, you can reclaim your energy, clarity, and resilience.

GLYPHOSATE—THE SILENT NUTRIENT THIEF

Glyphosate is the most widely used herbicide in the world. It's sprayed not just on GMO crops like corn and soy, but also on non-GMO grains (like wheat, oats, and barley) as a "drying agent" before harvest. That means even foods you wouldn't think of as "sprayed" can carry residues. It also contaminates water, soil, and even rainfall—so avoidance alone is nearly impossible.

Glyphosate's damage is subtle but far-reaching. It:

- ✓ Destroys gut bacteria, acting like a broad-spectrum antibiotic and wiping out beneficial microbes and allowing harmful ones to thrive.
- ✓ Blocks mineral absorption. Glyphosate binds to minerals like magnesium, zinc, and manganese, starving your cells of essential cofactors.
- ✓ Disrupts detox pathways. It inhibits enzymes in the liver that help clear toxins.
- ✓ Mimics glycine. This can interfere with protein synthesis and damage collagen, affecting joints, skin, and connective tissue.
- ✓ Contributes to leaky gut. It damages the tight junctions in the intestinal lining, increasing inflammation and auto-immune risk.

Common symptoms include digestive distress, bloating, nutrient deficiencies, joint pain, skin issues, fatigue, brain fog, hormonal imbalance, and increased autoimmune risk. Chronic exposure has been linked to infertility, kidney disease, neurological disorders, and even certain cancers.

COMMON SOURCES OF GLYPHOSATE

- Non-organic wheat, oats, barley, rye
- GMO soy, corn, canola
- Processed foods containing corn syrup, soy lecithin, or vegetable oils
- Conventionally raised animal products (via feed contamination)
- Beer, wine, and certain teas
- Even some supposedly "healthy" protein powders

DETOX STRATEGIES FOR GLYPHOSATE

1. Reduce ongoing exposure: Shift to organic whenever possible, especially for grains, beans, and animal products.

2. Support gut repair: L-glutamine, aloe vera, marshmallow root, and probiotics help restore the intestinal lining.

3. Bind and remove: Humic and fulvic acids, bentonite clay, and chlorella can help bind glyphosate. Some studies suggest certain probiotics (*Lactobacillus* strains) can break it down.

4. Mineral repletion: Focus on magnesium, zinc, and manganese to counter depletion.

5. Boost detox enzymes: Sulfur-rich foods (garlic, onions, broccoli sprouts) and compounds like NAC and milk thistle help reactivate the body's detox machinery.

6. Sweat and move: Exercise and sauna therapy encourage toxin release and circulation.

Glyphosate detox isn't just about removing a chemical—it's about restoring your body's ability to repair, absorb nutrients, and fight inflammation at its root.

Other Environmental Offenders			
Offenders	Source(s)	What They Do	Detox Strategies
fluoride & chlorine	tap water	neurotoxic in excess; impairs thyroid	reverse osmosis water, iodine-rich foods, boron, sauna, sweating, mineral repletion

microplastics & phthalates	bottled water, food packaging, cosmetics	disrupt hormones and gut	avoid plastic, sauna, fiber, chlorella, glutathione
PFAS ("forever chemicals")	nonstick cookware, waterproof fabrics, firefighting foam	linked to cancer, immune suppression	water filtration, sauna, bile-boosting foods, binders like activated charcoal
volatile organic compounds (VOCs)	off-gassing from furniture, paint, cleaning products	irritates lungs, damages mitochondria	air purifiers, indoor plants, regular ventilation, sweating, antioxidant support
endocrine-disrupting chemicals (EDCs)	BPA, parabens, triclosan; in plastics, personal care, receipts	disrupt hormones and fertility	swap to natural personal care, avoid canned foods, detox with cruciferous vegetables, sulforaphane, DIM

| food additives & artificial sweeteners | aspartame, MSG, dyes, emulsifiers | affect brain and gut | clean diet, probiotics, digestive enzymes, liver support |
| pesticides beyond glyphosate | organophosphates, neonicotinoids | harm nervous system | organic produce, washing/peeling, cilantro, chlorella, sauna |

DETOX IS NOT AN EVENT—IT'S A WAY OF LIFE

In a perfect world, detox wouldn't be necessary. But in *this* world—detox is no longer optional. It's a daily necessity, a form of cellular housekeeping that keeps your body resilient, your mind clear, and your spirit light. But here's the truth: You don't have to live in fear of toxins when you live in rhythm with your body, and you now have nine powerful detox strategies to help you do that! Each one is powerful on its own. But together, they create a lifestyle that continuously clears what does not belong so your energy, clarity, and healing potential can rise. The secret is in making detox a rhythm.

- » **Monthly**: Do a mini one-to-three day reset (soups, broths, herbal support).
- » **Seasonally**: Choose a deeper cleanse (e.g., spring = liver, fall = colon, winter = lymph, summer = spike detox).

- » **Daily**: Support the exits—sweat, move, hydrate, poop, breathe.
- » **Weekly**: Rebound, sauna, dry brush, castor oil pack.
- » **Yearly**: Cycle through all nine strategies across the year in a gentle, structured flow.

This keeps your body open, your terrain clear, and your health proactive, not reactive.

DR. LAURA'S PERSONAL RITUALS

These are the rhythms that keep me grounded, strong, and clear in a world that constantly pulls us off balance:

- ✓ Every morning, I drink warm lemon water with a pinch of air-dried sea salt and take one capsule of bentonite clay—before anything else.
- ✓ I do a liver and gallbladder flush every three months, always paired with a colonic to support elimination.
- ✓ I rebound every morning to wake up my lymphatic system and move my energy.
- ✓ I get natural sunlight on my skin and eyes every day—even just for a few minutes.
- ✓ I swim in the ocean whenever I can. Saltwater is medicine for the body and the spirit.
- ✓ I hike. I spend time in the forest. I touch the earth with my bare feet.
- ✓ And just as importantly, I spend time with positive, high-frequency humans—because your environment is part of your detox too.

This is not about being perfect. It's about staying connected—to the earth, to my body, and to the deeper rhythm of life. Now you have the tools. Use them often. Trust your body. Return to the wisdom of nature, and build a life that heals, one detox ritual at a time.

VIKING SUPERFOODS, HERBS, AND MODERN POWER NUTRIENTS —WHY ORDINARY FOOD IS NO LONGER ENOUGH

Let food be thy medicine—but let it be wild, wise, and worthy of your biology.

Twenty-first century Vikings are nutrient starved in a world of abundance, which is why eating clean isn't enough anymore. We've passed the point where kale salads and green smoothies can fix it all: Our soil is depleted, because modern farming strips it of minerals like magnesium, iodine, and selenium. Our water is filtered, fluoridated, and sterilized—and void of trace minerals. Most people eat processed, plastic-wrapped, ultra-heated, chemically sprayed food. And even healthy eaters are often deficient in omega-3s, vitamin D, magnesium, B12, and iodine. Plus, the body is under constant assault from pesticides and other toxins. To thrive in this era, modern Vikings must fuel themselves with superfoods.

Superfoods are not a trend. They are the concentrated nutritional forces that can rebuild what modern life has stripped away. They provide high-density vitamins and minerals in absorbable forms; antioxidants that neutralize oxidative damage from pollution and radiation; detox compounds that bind and eliminate toxins from the liver, gut, and brain; and adaptogens and phytochemicals that restore resilience, hormone balance, and immune strength.

THIS IS NUTRITIONAL SURVIVAL

This isn't about trendy powders or fads. This is about survival in a toxic world. Every meal becomes an opportunity to defend, rebuild, and recharge your cells. To be strong, sharp, and sovereign in the twenty-first century, you need to fortify your body like a warrior—with foods and compounds that heal you at the cellular level. To eat like a modern Viking is to fight back. Every bite becomes your weapon. Every meal becomes your medicine. And your vitality becomes your revolution.

VIKING-ERA SUPERFOODS AND FORGOTTEN PLANT ALLIES

These foods and herbs were likely a part of the Viking landscape—and they still pack a punch today.

As discussed on page 6, **wild fish** and **roe** are rich in the essential omega-3s, DHA and EPA. Fish roe (like salmon eggs and cod liver) is also high in phospholipids, choline, zinc, vitamin D, and vitamin A—nutrients essential for fertility, immunity, and strong development. These foods were prized by coastal cultures for vitality and resilience. *Eat wild salmon, sardines, mackerel, herring, cod liver, and caviar.*

Chaga mushrooms are known as the King of Medicinal Mushrooms in Nordic and Baltic traditions. Chaga is loaded with betulinic acid, polysaccharides, and melanin-rich antioxidants that support liver detox, cellular protection, immune modulation, and gut lining repair. *Drink as a slow-simmered tea, tincture, or dual extract powder.*

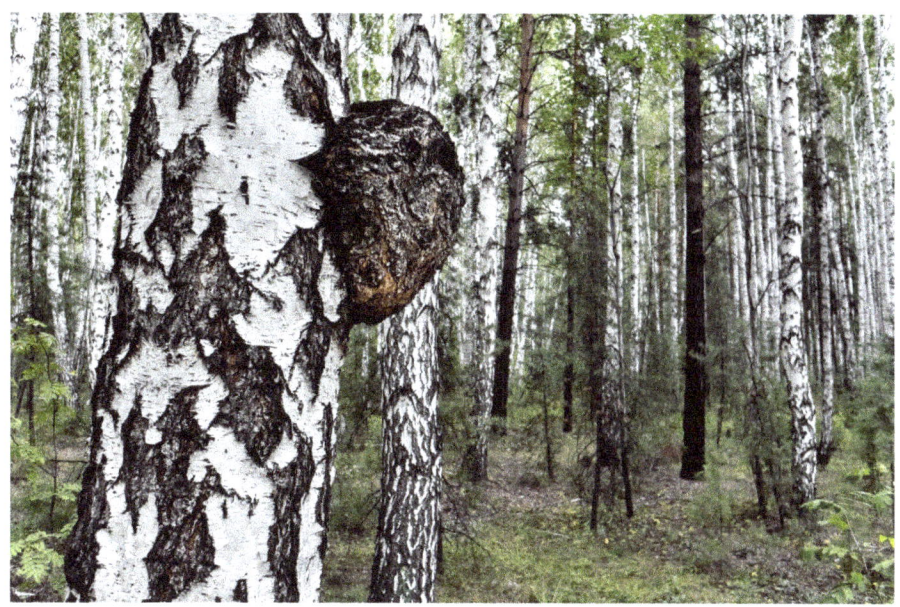

Vikings brewed mead—a fermented honey wine—which was valued for its rejuvenating properties and spiritual significance. **Raw honey** itself is antimicrobial, antioxidant, and wound-healing, while **bee pollen** contains every essential amino acid, along with enzymes, minerals, and B vitamins. Together, they're powerful tonics for energy, immunity, and gut health. *Use raw local honey and bee pollen in smoothies or on fruit.*

An often-overlooked weed, **nettle** is loaded with nutrients, making it a natural blood builder. Its histamine-modulating properties support joint health and seasonal allergy relief. *Use as tea, tincture, soup green, or dry-leaf powder.*

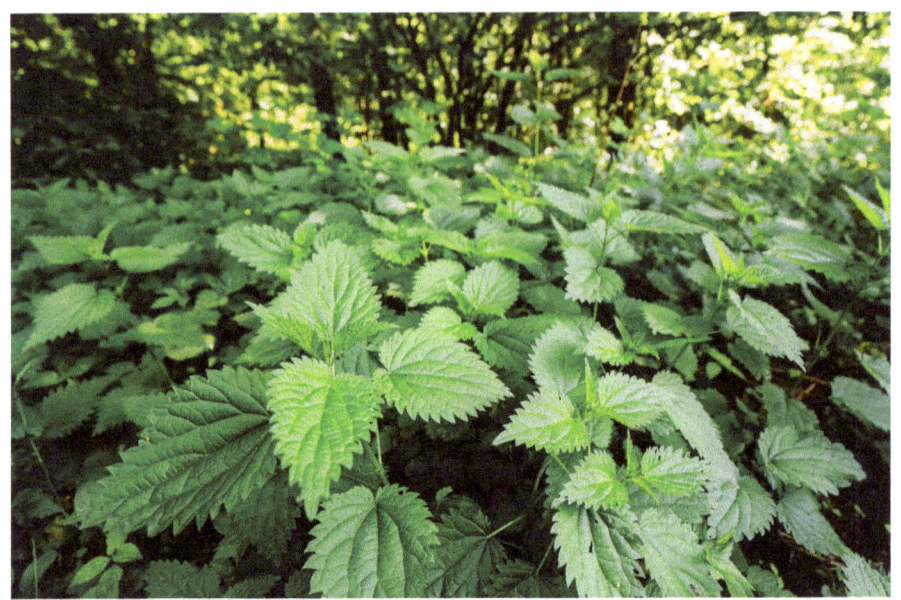

Bilberries, lingonberries, and **cloudberries** support vascular health, eye function, and reduce oxidative stress—especially bilberries, which are used in modern formulas for vision support. Their deep pigments signal powerful immune and anti-aging benefits. *Eat fresh, dried, or freeze-dried powder in smoothies or yogurt.*

Both **dandelion root** and **leaf** are deeply cleansing and stimulate bile flow, liver detox, and kidney drainage, making them a gentle daily tonic for purification. They also support skin clarity and gut motility—perfect for spring cleansing or daily balance. *Use as a tea, roasted root coffee alternative, or fresh leaf in salads.*

Garlic is a natural antibiotic, antiviral, and antiparasitic—used since ancient times to protect and purify the body. **Wild garlic** is even more potent and is often infused into oils or vinegars. Vikings also relied on **fermented foods** like cabbage (sauerkraut), fish (rakfisk), and dairy (kefir-like drinks) as key sources of probiotics and digestive enzymes. *Use fresh garlic daily, and include fermented veggies or drinks with meals.*

MODERN NUTRIENT WARRIORS FOR THE TWENTY-FIRST CENTURY

Below are the essential nutrients and compounds your modern body is often missing.

Magnesium (glycinate, malate, or threonate) is involved in over 300 enzymatic reactions in the body, yet it's chronically depleted by stress, caffeine, sugar, and modern farming. It calms the nervous system, relaxes tight muscles, supports detoxification pathways, and improves sleep quality. Use glycinate for calm, malate for energy, and threonate for brain health—especially during stressful or cleansing phases.

Omega-3 **DHA** is vital for cognitive clarity and mood, whereas **EPA** regulates inflammation and hormone balance. Choose a clean algae-based DHA (for its purity and sustainability), and pair it with tocotrienol-rich vitamin E for enhanced absorption and cellular protection.

Shilajit is a tar-like adaptogen sourced from ancient mountain ranges—formed from compressed plant matter over thousands of years. It delivers over 80 trace minerals, along with fulvic acid to help shuttle nutrients into your cells and remove waste. Shilajit has been shown to increase mitochondrial function, enhance testosterone, and support cognitive and detox capacity.

CoQ10 and **PQQ** work together to supercharge your cellular energy. CoQ10 is essential for mitochondrial ATP production and helps protect the heart, brain, and muscles, especially as we age.

PQQ not only supports mitochondrial function but also stimulates the growth of new mitochondria—a rare and powerful effect known as mitochondrial biogenesis.

Glutathione is the body's most powerful antioxidant, defending against free radicals, environmental toxins, and cellular damage. **NAC** (N-acetylcysteine) helps your body naturally produce more glutathione, especially during illness, stress, or toxin exposure. Together, they protect the liver, lungs, and brain—making them essential for detox, immune defense, and long-term vitality.

Adaptogens help your body adapt to physical, emotional, and environmental stressors by balancing cortisol and supporting adrenal health. **Ashwagandha** calms anxiety and supports thyroid function; **rhodiola** boosts endurance and mood; **holy basil** soothes inflammation; and **eleuthero** enhances stamina and resilience. Use during burnout, recovery, hormonal imbalances, or whenever life feels overwhelming.

Lion's mane stimulates nerve growth factor (NGF), aiding in brain regeneration, memory, and mental clarity. **Reishi**, revered as the "mushroom of immortality," helps regulate immune function, calm the nervous system, and support restful sleep and detox. These medicinal fungi are ancient allies for modern stress, brain health, and immune resilience.

Zinc, iodine, boron, and **selenium** are essential for hormone production, thyroid balance, fertility, immunity, and detoxification. Modern farming, processed foods, and filtered water have stripped these from our diets, leaving many people deficient. Replenish through sea vegetables (like kelp or dulse), mineral drops, or whole-food supplements to restore what your cells need to thrive.

A word on **supplements**: They should supplement nature, not replace it. When choosing supplements, buy natural and organic whenever possible. Look for supplements that are in their full-spectrum, food-based, or bioavailable form, and delivered in liquid, powder, or clean capsules (no tablets or soft gels). Seek out supplements with veggie capsules—no fillers, flowing agents, or hidden excipients—from companies that practice transparency and integrity. Avoid magnesium stearate, silicon dioxide, titanium dioxide, and artificial colors or preservatives. Your supplements should be clean enough to eat—and wise enough to work.

BUILD YOUR WARRIOR'S PANTRY

Imagine a shelf in your kitchen stocked with:

- Grass-fed liver capsules (liver health)
- Raw honey and bee pollen (immunity and gut health)
- Fermented foods alive with probiotics (gut health)
- Seaweed for your soup (iodine, minerals, and cellular hydration)
- Chaga for your tea (immune intelligence)
- Wild berries for your breakfast (brain protection)
- Dandelion, nettle, and arugula for your salads (liver-cleansing greens)
- Bone broth with mushrooms, miso, or garlic (gut healing and immune modulation)
- Spirulina, chlorella, shilajit, or fulvic minerals for your smoothies (bind and clear toxins)
- Raw pumpkin seeds or Brazil nuts for snacks (zinc and selenium)
- Omega-3s from algae oil or wild fish (brain, hormones, and inflammation control)

- This isn't about pills. It's about reclaiming vitality from the earth and sea—just like your ancestors did.

DR. LAURA'S TOP FIVE DAILY MUST-HAVES

1. Omega-3s EPA/DHA are foundational for brain, heart, nerves, and cellular repair.

2. Minerals: Magnesium and iodine are critical for thousands of cell functions.

3. B complex and D3 and K2 for energy, hormones, immunity, and calcium metabolism

4. Digestive enzymes for gut health, nutrient absorption, and inflammation control.

5. Delta tocotrienols are powerful fat-soluble antioxidants that protect your cells from EMFs, radiation, and chemical toxicity.

DAILY RITUALS OF THE MODERN VIKING

"Travel light, live light, spread the light, and be light." –Yogi Bhajan

The Vikings didn't separate "self-care" from survival. Every breath, every movement, every bite, every fire lit, and water drawn was done with intention. Their entire life was a ritual.

If you want Viking-level strength in today's world, you have to move with purpose, train your mind, engage your spirit, sweat out the toxins, sharpen your edges, and reconnect to what's real. This chapter is your blueprint for how to live like a Viking in the twenty-first century—even if you're in a city, working full-time, and surrounded by modern chaos.

MORNING AWAKENING RITUAL

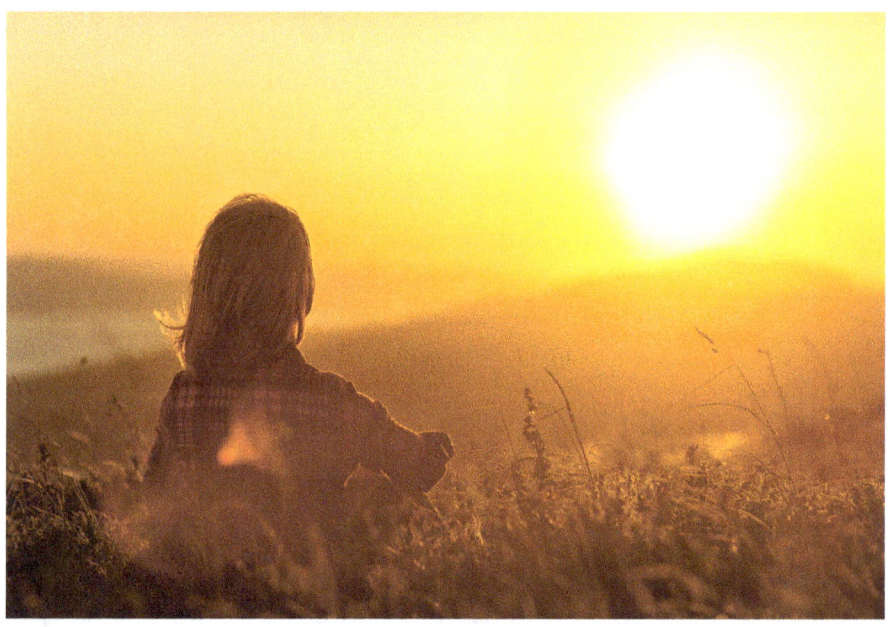

Vikings didn't hit snooze. They woke up with the sun and prepared for battle—whether that battle was farming, fishing, hunting, or surviving the cold.

Your modern ritual: Wake with the sun or within 30 minutes of sunrise. Step outside immediately—barefoot if possible—and face the light. This resets your circadian rhythm and boosts dopamine. Drink 16–24 oz. of warm water with lemon, minerals, or ACV to flush and hydrate. Breathe deeply, stretch, and set your mind for the day like a warrior sharpening a blade. Even 10 minutes of morning connection sets the tone for everything.

BREATH WORK AND COLD EXPOSURE

Vikings weren't afraid of the cold. The cold made them stronger. Modern studies now confirm that cold + breath work = mitochondrial magic. It boosts brown fat and supports detox pathways, immunity, metabolism, and mental clarity.

Your modern ritual: Take cold showers (start warm, end cold for 30–60 seconds). Partake in ice baths or cold plunges 2–3 times per week if available, for 1–3 minutes—but don't overdo it, especially women. Practice Wim Hof breathing, box breathing, or deep nasal breathing. Combine it all with nature: cold + breath + forest = instant nervous system reset. Cold makes you resilient. Breath makes you present. Together, they rewire your biology.

FUNCTIONAL MOVEMENT AND WARRIOR TRAINING

Vikings didn't do bicep curls. They carried wood, rowed boats, climbed rocks, and wrestled their kin. Your body was designed to move, lift, stretch, hang, squat, crawl, sprint, and recover.

Your modern ritual: Walk 5,000–10,000 steps per day—non-negotiable. Lift something heavy 2–4x/week (weights, kettlebells, logs, kids). Sprint, row, bike, or do HIIT-style cardio 1–2x/week. Stretch, hang from a bar, foam roll, or do mobility daily. Train outside whenever possible—sunlight and grounding is performance fuel.

MENTAL DISCIPLINE AND INNER FORTITUDE

The greatest warriors didn't just train the body—they mastered the mind. Vikings believed in fate, in honor, and in legacy. They didn't waste time on drama, doubt, or distraction. That's your challenge today—cut through the noise and strengthen your inner world.

Your modern ritual: Journal daily—even just three lines of truth. Practice 5-10 minutes of stillness (meditation, prayer, silence). Read something that makes you wiser, and limit toxic media—especially in the morning. Speak less, listen more, observe your reactions; inner strength is quiet, but it radiates.

SAUNA, SWEAT, AND DETOX RITUALS

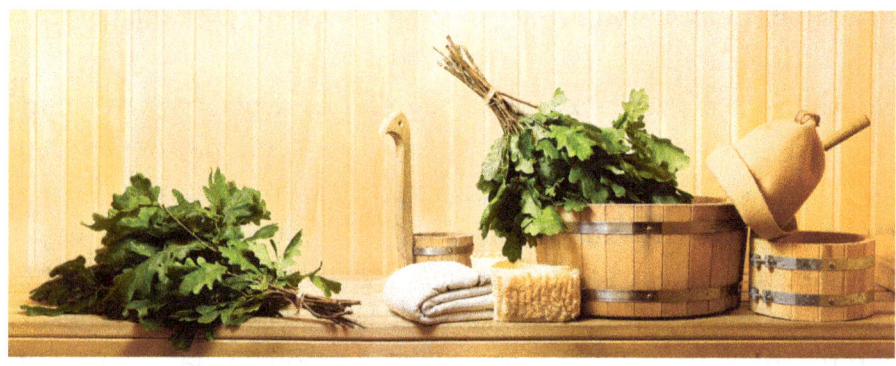

The sauna was the original Viking wellness tool. In fact, "sweat lodge" culture was common in the Nordic and Baltic worlds. Today, science has proven that regular sweating reduces all-cause mortality, improves circulation, purges toxins, and boosts resilience.

Your modern ritual: Use an infrared or traditional sauna 3-5 times per week (even 15-20 minutes is gold). Follow with cold (shower, plunge, or fresh air). Be sure to dry brush beforehand to stimulate lymph flow. Drink electrolytes, take binders if detoxing, and rest afterward. Sweating is your body's built-in release valve. Use it often.

NIGHTFALL GROUNDING RITUAL

Vikings honored the fire at night—gathering, reflecting, resting. In our world of blue light, stress, and artificial stimulation, your evening ritual is how you close the loop and reset the nervous system.

Your modern ritual: Power down screens one hour before sleep. Light a candle, fire, or use low red lighting. Read, stretch, pray, or journal, and take a calming tea: chamomile, reishi, lemon balm, passionflower. Sleep 7–9 hrs. in total darkness. Sleep is your regeneration cycle—where hormones are balanced, the brain is washed, and healing happens.

BONUS: WEEKLY SACRED PRACTICES

- Forest bathing (get into the woods)
- Fasting (12–16 hrs. or one- or two-meal days)
- Digital detox days
- Sun gazing at sunrise or sunset
- Community gatherings or meals with loved ones
- Cold plunges in natural water. If you can find it, do it

You don't need to live in a longhouse or wear animal pelts to live like a Viking. You just need to show up—daily—with intention, reverence, and strength. Live by ritual. Train your mind, move your body, feed your soul—and become the kind of human the modern world desperately needs: clear, grounded, resilient, and free.

RECAPTURING CALM—THE VIKING MINDSET AND EMOTIONAL RESILIENCE

You can drink green juice, take all the right supplements, and detox your cells—but if your spirit is fragmented, your healing will stall.

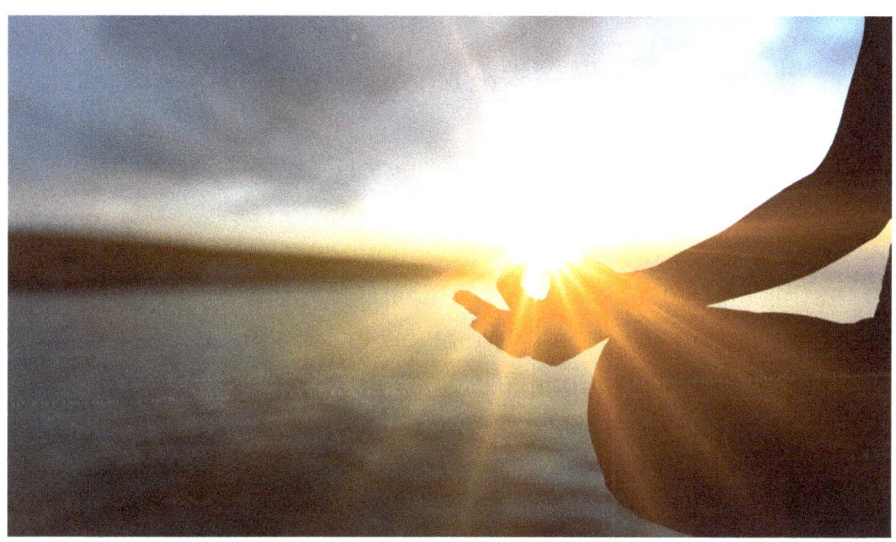

The Vikings were survivors of famine, plague, bitter cold, and devastating loss. They knew hardship—but they also knew how to transmute it. They wept and warred. They prayed and persevered. And in their strength, we find a blueprint.

This chapter isn't about pretending life is easy; it's about choosing to rise anyway. While we're not running from wild beasts today, we are *drowning* in digital overstimulation, emotional fragmentation, and relentless noise. Our nervous systems weren't designed for this level of chronic activation.

WHAT STRESS DOES TO THE BODY

- Activates the sympathetic nervous system (fight-or-flight)
- Triggers the release of cortisol and adrenaline
- Suppresses digestion, hormone production, and immune function
- Inhibits the vagus nerve—cutting off calm, healing, and connection
- Disrupts sleep, increases blood sugar, and slows detox pathways
- Shrinks the hippocampus (memory center) and weakens emotional regulation

In this state, the body cannot heal. It's too busy surviving. You could be eating the cleanest diet on Earth—but if your body is stuck in fight-or-flight, your cells won't absorb nutrients. Your detox organs won't release waste. Your hormones won't balance. Your brain won't regenerate.

FROM SCIENCE TO STRATEGY: WHAT HELPS US SHIFT

You don't have to eliminate all stress—but you do need to shift your baseline. You must teach your body how to feel safe again. Here's what works—backed by both science and ancient wisdom:

1. Regulate your nervous system—Breath work activates the vagus nerve and reduces cortisol. Cold exposure increases stress resilience and dopamine. Grounding (barefoot on Earth) restores circadian rhythm and reduces inflammation. Rebounding or light movement flushes lymph and calms the mind. *Practice*: box breathing (4-4-4-4); 30-second cold showers; walking barefoot in the grass, forest, or beach (10+ minutes/day).

2. Rewire your inner voice—The subconscious listens. Every word you speak to yourself becomes a command to your body. Science shows that self-talk affects the limbic system, shaping your emotions, immune response, and even physical recovery. *Practice*: Replace "Why is this happening to me?" with "What is this teaching me?" or "I am being refined—not broken."

3. Clean up your input—Your mind is a garden; what you consume becomes your soil. The nervous system is always listening, even to background news, social media, and noise. Over time, this creates chronic low-level fear and cortisol elevation. *Practice*: Curate your feed; turn off notifications; take one digital detox day per week; spend time with people who energize, not drain.

4. Process, don't suppress—Suppressed emotion becomes stagnation. Grief becomes gut tension. Anger becomes liver heat. Fear settles into the kidneys. The Vikings didn't bottle it up; they sang, wept, screamed, and danced around fires. *Practice*: journal raw emotions; cry in the car; scream into a pillow; dance to drumbeats; sweat it out.

5. Anchor into a bigger story—You are not your diagnosis. You are not your bank account, your trauma, or your pain. You are part of a longer, deeper story—of warriors, healers, mothers, survivors. Science confirms that a sense of purpose, identity, and ancestral belonging improves resilience, immunity, and even longevity. *Practice*: Say aloud, "What would the strongest version of me do today?" or "My ancestors overcame more than this."

Below are some additional emotional detox tools for the modern Viking to help reduce stress and promote healing and abundance.

- ✓ Nature immersion: forest, mountain, ocean
- ✓ Smudging with pine, sage, or mugwort
- ✓ Saying "no" to energy leaks
- ✓ Saying "yes" to joy, creation, and laughter
- ✓ Digital sabbaticals
- ✓ Spiritual rituals, prayer, and ancestral connection
- ✓ Repeat modern Viking affirmations every day. (Speak them out loud. Let your body hear them.)

Remember, your mind is the battlefield. You are not broken; you are being reshaped! You are returning to something ancient inside you. This is not toxic positivity. This is sacred reclamation. You are becoming the warrior your lineage has been waiting for.

AFFIRMATIONS

MORNING

I am clear.
I am strong.
I am grounded in truth.
I rise with courage.
I walk with wisdom.
I am the architect of my day.

EVENING

I release what no longer belongs to me.
I trust the rhythm of my breath.
I surrender to rest.
I am safe, I am guided, I am enough.
Tomorrow will meet me in strength.

THE LONGEVITY CODE—ANCIENT WISDOM MEETS MODERN SCIENCE

Live long—and live well.

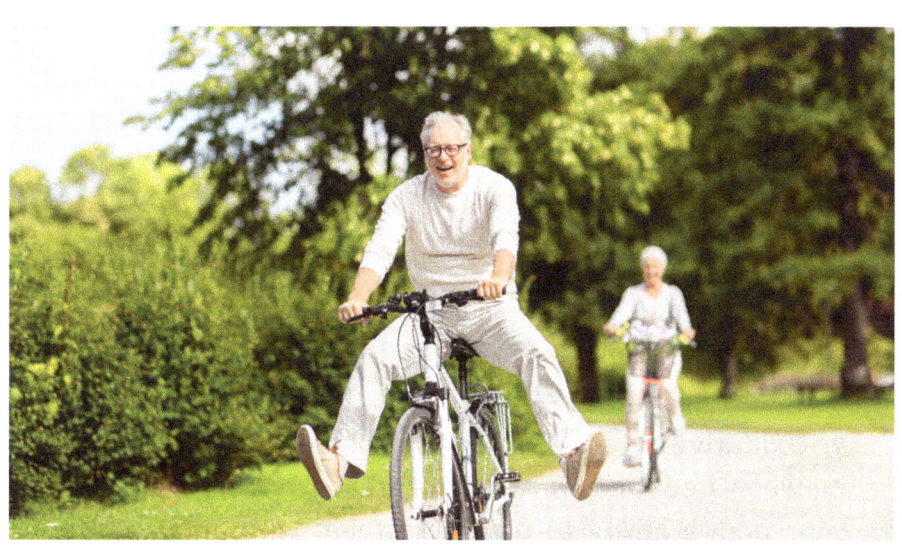

What if aging was optional—or at least how fast we age?

For centuries, humans believed that aging was a slow, inevitable decline. But across the world—from the mountain monks of China to the centenarians of the Mediterranean—there have always been whispers of those who defied time. And now, in the twenty-first century, the science is beginning to catch up with the secrets.

We're living in the golden age of longevity research. One of the pioneers, who truly understood both the mystical and the molecular sides of aging, is David Avocado Wolfe, whose *Longevity Now* philosophy blended superfoods, detoxification, and joyful living into a practical path for vibrant health.

As a doctor of Chinese medicine with a foundation in clinical work, energetic medicine, and years of treating real people, I've witnessed something powerful: True longevity isn't about chasing youth. It's about becoming more alive, more vital, and more connected—with every passing year. It's not about how much time you can squeeze out of life. It's about how much vitality you can bring into it.

Let's explore what modern science and ancient wisdom both tell us about how to live not just longer, but better.

WHAT'S ACTUALLY AGING US?

Modern research has identified six key drivers of aging—processes that wear down the body over time.

1. Oxidative stress happens when there's an imbalance between free radicals—unstable, reactive molecules—and your body's ability to neutralize them with antioxidants. Free radicals "steal" electrons from healthy cells, damaging cell membranes, DNA, proteins, and mitochondria. This accelerates aging at the cellular level and is linked to everything from wrinkles and fatigue to cancer and heart disease.

What to do about it:

- » Eat antioxidant-rich foods (berries, turmeric, dark leafy greens, cacao).
- » Take glutathione, vitamin C, alpha lipoic acid, and delta tocotrienols.
- » Avoid smoking, processed food, and environmental toxins.
- » Reduce EMF exposure and blue light at night.
- » Fast occasionally to stimulate internal antioxidant systems (like NRF2 pathway).

2. Chronic inflammation is a low-grade fire that fuels all disease. Although inflammation itself is your body's defense system, when it stays activated—due to toxins, infections, stress, or poor diet—it becomes chronic, silently damaging tissues and aging your body from the inside out.

Chronic inflammation is behind nearly every modern disease: heart disease, cancer, diabetes, Alzheimer's, autoimmune disorders, and even depression. It also disrupts hormones, collagen production, and brain function.

What to do about it:

- » Adopt an anti-inflammatory diet (omega-3s, wild herbs, low sugar).
- » Avoid processed foods, seed oils, and artificial ingredients.
- » Use herbs like turmeric, boswellia, ginger, and reishi.
- » Heal the gut (70 percent of immune activity originates here).
- » Incorporate movement, cold exposure, and breath work to regulate inflammation naturally.

3. Telomere shortening: Telomeres are protective caps at the ends of your DNA. Every time your cells divide, telomeres get shorter—eventually leading to cellular aging and death.

Short telomeres are linked to aging, decreased lifespan, heart disease, immune decline, and cellular instability. They're like the plastic tips on shoelaces—once they wear out, the entire strand unravels.

What to do about it:

- » Use Astragalus extract (TA-65) to support telomerase, the enzyme that rebuilds telomeres.
- » Practice meditation and stress reduction (stress rapidly shortens telomeres).
- » Exercise moderately (especially walking, rebounding, resistance training).
- » Eat a nutrient-dense, antioxidant-rich diet.
- » Avoid smoking, poor sleep, and excess alcohol.

4. Mitochondrial decline: Mitochondria are the "batteries" of your cells—producing over 90 percent of your body's energy (ATP). As we age, mitochondrial function declines due to oxidative damage, toxins, and nutrient depletion.

When your mitochondria weaken, so does everything else: brain fog, fatigue, muscle loss, hormone issues, and aging skin. It's like powering a city on a dying generator.

What to do about it:

- » Take CoQ10 (ubiquinol) and PQQ to protect and generate new mitochondria.
- » Use shilajit and magnesium malate to fuel mitochondrial activity.

- » Do high-intensity interval training (HIIT) and cold exposure to stimulate biogenesis.
- » Avoid toxins (plastics, heavy metals, pesticides) that damage mitochondria.
- » Support detox with glutathione, alpha lipoic acid, and fasting.

5. Senescent cells are damaged, dysfunctional cells that no longer divide—but they don't die. They sit in tissues and release inflammatory substances that damage surrounding cells. Known as "zombie cells," they promote aging and disease.

Senescent cells fuel low-grade inflammation (inflammaging), accelerate tissue breakdown, and impair organ function. They're linked to arthritis, neurodegeneration, cardiovascular disease, and skin aging.

What to do about it:

- » Use fisetin (found in strawberries) and quercetin to clear senescent cells.
- » Incorporate 24-to-72-hr. fasting to trigger autophagy (cell cleanup).
- » Take curcumin, resveratrol, and EGCG to reduce senescent cell signals.
- » Exercise and stay lean—fat tissue harbors more senescent cells.
- » Consider senolytics (compounds that selectively remove these cells) in supervised protocols.

6. Glycation happens when sugar molecules bind to proteins or fats, creating sticky compounds called advanced glycation end products (AGEs). These damage tissues, stiffen collagen, and accelerate aging.

AGEs contribute to skin sagging, arterial stiffness, kidney decline, and insulin resistance. They also inflame the brain, leading to cognitive issues. Glycation is especially accelerated in diabetics and high-carb diets.

What to do about it:

» Cut excess sugar and refined carbs.
» Avoid charred and fried foods (they're loaded with AGEs).
» Take carnosine, alpha-lipoic acid, and benfotiamine—powerful antiglycation nutrients.
» Eat plenty of antioxidants to reduce the oxidative stress that worsens glycation.
» Fast intermittently to lower blood sugar and insulin.

Each of these six drivers may sound separate—but they're deeply interconnected.

For example: Oxidative stress causes mitochondrial damage. Mitochondrial damage increases inflammation. Inflammation speeds up senescence and telomere loss. The good news? We can slow—and in some cases, reverse—these processes.

True longevity requires a multi-layered strategy—one that addresses root causes, not just symptoms. And that's exactly what *The Modern Viking Diet* is designed to do.

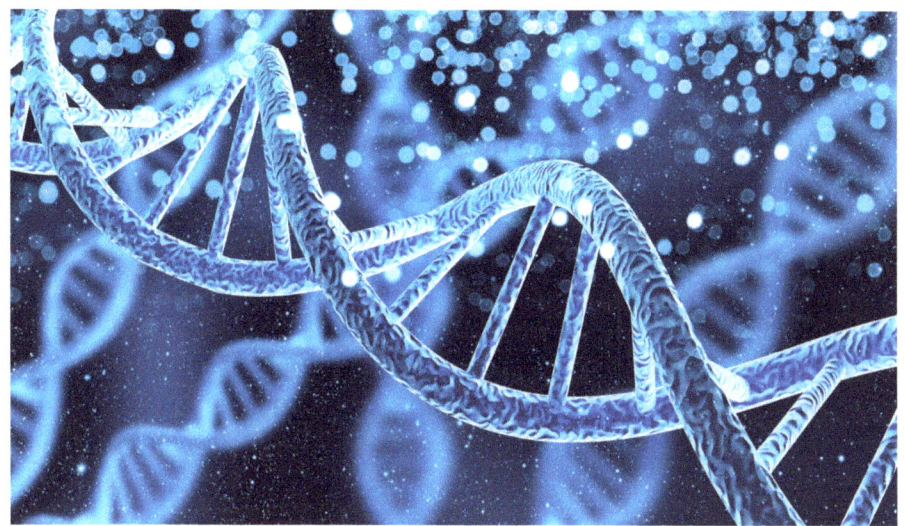

YOUR LONGEVITY BLUEPRINT

One of the most powerful yet overlooked approaches to longevity blends ancient herbalism with modern cellular science—not through trends or extremes, but through nature's built-in intelligence. This philosophy centers around the idea that true vitality is not about suppressing aging but about activating the body's natural capacity to regenerate. It begins with **hormetic stressors**—brief, intentional challenges like cold exposure, sauna, or fasting—that nudge the body into resilience mode, switching on repair pathways that lie dormant in our comfort-driven world. These practices are paired with **superfoods** and **tonic herbs** that have been used for centuries to nourish *Jing* (core essence), support adrenal and immune function, and enhance cellular detoxification.

Another key focus is **enzyme therapy**, which clears undigested proteins, scar tissue, and toxic residues that accumulate over time.

It's internal maintenance at the cellular level—sweeping the debris that blocks energy and healing. This internal cleanup sets the stage for regeneration.

Perhaps most crucially, this system aims to reduce **calcification** (rigid tissues due to mineral imbalance) and **glycation** (sugar-damaged proteins), two often-ignored but major contributors to premature aging. It also emphasizes clearing senescent cells, the cells that linger in the body long after their purpose is gone, releasing inflammatory signals that damage nearby healthy cells.

The core belief is simple: When you **upgrade your internal terrain**—your biological soil—disease cannot take root, energy flows freely, and longevity becomes a natural result of deep nourishment. This is not just a health plan; it's a way of honoring your cells with the conditions they need to thrive. Let me expand on some of these approaches.

HORMETIC STRESS

The human body wasn't designed for constant comfort. In fact, some of the most potent longevity triggers are activated not by supplements—but by brief, controlled stress.

> **Cold exposure**, such as cold plunges, ocean swims, or even finishing your shower with 30 seconds of icy water, activates brown fat and stimulates mitochondrial activity. This, in turn, boosts metabolism, mental clarity, and immune defense. The Vikings likely practiced this unknowingly—jumping into frigid fjords after sweating in fire-warmed huts. Today, science confirms it: Cold exposure increases norepinephrine,

reduces inflammation, and stimulates resilience at the cellular level.

Sauna therapy, especially infrared or traditional wood-fired, works at the opposite end of the hormetic spectrum. Deep heat activates heat shock proteins, which repair damaged proteins in the body, aid in detoxification, and protect against neurodegeneration. Saunas also mimic exercise by increasing heart rate, blood circulation, and lymphatic flow—all while promoting calm through endorphin release. Studies have linked regular sauna use to lower risk of cardiovascular disease, dementia, and all-cause mortality.

Fasting—whether intermittent (like 16:8), time-restricted, or occasional 24-to-72-hour fasts—gives your body a break from constant digestion and instead activates autophagy, the process by which cells clear out damaged components. Fasting reduces insulin resistance, lowers inflammation, and triggers the release of human growth hormone (HGH)—all crucial for repair and longevity. In ancient cultures, fasting wasn't a diet trend; it was built into the natural rhythm of scarcity, travel, and spiritual rituals.

Together, these three forms of hormetic stress act as biological "tune-ups"—helping the body stay young by challenging it just enough to spark adaptation.

TONIC HERBS AND SUPERFOODS: NATURE'S CODE FOR REGENERATION

Long before modern medicine, cultures around the world relied on tonic herbs—not just to fight disease but also to enhance vitality. These herbs were seen as longevity elixirs, often reserved for royalty, warriors, or the elders of the tribe.

He shou wu (fo-ti) is a revered herb in Chinese medicine for restoring *Jing*. It's known to support the kidneys, hair, reproductive function, and cellular regeneration. Stories tell of ancient sages using it to extend life, and modern science shows it has antioxidant and neuroprotective effects.

Reishi mushrooms have been used for centuries to calm the spirit, support the immune system, and balance the nervous system. They are especially helpful in modulating stress responses, improving sleep, and reducing inflammation—all pillars of longevity.

Chaga mushrooms support DNA repair, immunity, and gut integrity. They also protect against oxidative stress and help regulate blood sugar.

Astragalus is a powerful adaptogen that not only strengthens the immune system but also contains compounds like TA-65, believed to support telomerase activity—the enzyme that protects telomeres. By preserving telomere length, astragalus may help slow the biological clock.

Superfoods like wild berries, sea buckthorn, and AFA blue-green algae complement these herbs by flooding the body with bioavailable nutrients—micronutrients that many modern diets lack due to soil depletion. The goal is not just nourishment, but also cellular reactivation.

ENZYME THERAPY: THE FORGOTTEN KEY TO CELLULAR CLEANUP

Most people don't realize that by the time we reach our forties, our enzyme production declines dramatically. Enzymes are the microscopic machines that run nearly every function in the body: digestion, energy production, detoxification, and immune regulation. When undigested proteins and metabolic waste build up, inflammation and aging accelerate.

Proteolytic enzymes like serrapeptase, nattokinase, and bromelain break down fibrin (a protein involved in scar tissue and blood clots), helping to clear out stagnation and support clean blood flow. These enzymes are especially effective when taken on an empty stomach, as they bypass digestion and go directly into systemic circulation.

THE SILENT WRECKING CREW

Two of the most destructive and least discussed aging processes are **calcification** and **glycation**. Calcification occurs when calcium is deposited in soft tissues where it doesn't belong—like arteries, joints, pineal glands, and even the brain. It's often due to imbalanced magnesium levels or a lack of vitamin K2, which is critical for directing calcium into bones instead of blood vessels. Calcification contributes to arthritis, arterial stiffness, and decreased brain function. Glycation, on the other hand, leads to stiffness, wrinkles, loss of elasticity in blood vessels, and oxidative stress.

You can fight these processes by:

- ✓ Limiting sugar and ultra-processed food
- ✓ Using magnesium, vitamin K2, and tocotrienols (a potent form of vitamin E)
- ✓ Eating antioxidants from berries, herbs, and greens
- ✓ Incorporating fasting and enzymes to clear damaged cells

UPGRADING THE INTERNAL TERRAIN: REGENERATION OVER RESTRICTION

The most powerful longevity strategy isn't restriction—it's **restoration**. When you create a biological landscape that's clean, hydrated, mineral-rich, and energized, your cells will do what they were designed to do: repair and thrive.

This means supporting:

- Your detox organs: especially liver, kidneys, lymph, and skin
- Your mitochondria: with CoQ10, PQQ, and cold exposure
- Your microbiome: with fiber, prebiotics, probiotics, and fermented foods
- Your hormonal system: with adaptogens, healthy fats, and rhythmic living
- Your nervous system: through emotional resilience, sleep, and breath work

Longevity isn't just a number—it's a frequency. It's how your body feels when you wake up, how fast your wounds heal, how clear your mind is after fasting, how easily you laugh, and how deeply you sleep. It's not about chasing youth—it's about amplifying vital force.

When you upgrade your terrain—when you treat your inner ecosystem like sacred land—you unlock the true blueprint of health that has always been encoded in your cells.

OTHER SUPERFOODS OF THE FUTURE —AND THE PAST

AFA (Aphanizomenon flos-aquae) is a rare blue-green algae that may be the most nutrient-dense food on the planet. It's loaded with chlorophyll, trace minerals, and phenylethylamine (PEA)—a natural compound linked to joy, focus, and emotional resilience. It also contains compounds that support stem cell migration, cellular repair, and neural regeneration.

Omega-3 DHA isn't just a "good fat," it reduces inflammation at the root of chronic disease. It even correlates with longer telomeres—the biological markers of youth. People with higher DHA levels have lower risks of mortality from all causes. It's not just a supplement—it's a lifespan amplifier.

Sea buckthorn, a bright orange berry, is a powerhouse of omega-7s, vitamin C, and flavonoids. It repairs skin and mucous membranes, supports the gut lining, and nourishes the cardiovascular system. Traditionally used to heal wounds, today it's a modern anti-aging gem for inflammation, collagen, and metabolic health.

Aloe vera was once called the "plant of immortality" by ancient Egyptians. It supports detox pathways, heals the gut lining, and contains acemannan, a rare polysaccharide that may stimulate stem cells and immune regeneration.

Glutathione is the master antioxidant system of your body. It defends against free radicals, clears heavy metals, supports mitochondria, and even helps protect telomeres. **NAC** (N-acetyl cysteine) is the precursor that helps you make more glutathione naturally.

Quercetin and **fisetin** are *senolytics*—plant compounds that help your body clear out senescent cells (those cells that no longer function but cause harm). When you reduce senescent cell burden, you improve tissue regeneration, reduce inflammation, and protect against age-related decline.

PQQ (Pyrroloquinoline quinone) is like a fertilizer for your mitochondria. It triggers mitochondrial biogenesis, creating new energy-producing cells. PQQ sharpens cognition, improves stamina, and buffers the effects of oxidative stress.

MODERN ANTI-AGING TOOLS

There are plenty of other things—that will cost you nothing—to help you combat the aging process. **Exercise**, for example, turns on longevity genes like AMPK and SIRT1. Resistance training preserves mitochondrial density and muscle (key in aging), and walking increases blood flow to the brain and gut. Just 15 minutes a day can extend your health span.

Fasting is another option. It's not starvation, it's cellular optimization. Intermittent fasting (like 16:8 or 18:6) switches on autophagy—your body's cellular cleanup crew. Longer fasts under supervision can reset the immune system and rejuvenate stem cells. As we age, our need for frequent eating declines. Fasting becomes a fountain of youth.

Prioritize **deep sleep**. Sleep is when your body heals, rewires the brain, and resets your hormones. Melatonin—produced only in deep darkness—is a powerful antioxidant and DNA repair molecule. Sleep helps regulate inflammation, balance blood sugar, and protect telomeres.

Learn to **manage stress** like a master. Stress is one of the fastest ways to age your body. Cortisol burns through hormones, nutrients, and brain tissue. Breath work, cold plunges, and grounding reset the nervous system. Joy, laughter, music, and spiritual connection raise your vibration and longevity potential.

Then there are the ancient longevity practices that are still valid today. While Western science is just catching up, ancient systems like Traditional Chinese Medicine, Ayurveda, and Indigenous Earth Medicine always prioritized life extension through balance. **Tonic herbs** like astragalus, reishi, he shou wu, and ginseng were used to preserve *Jing*—your essence. **Seasonal cleansing** supported natural cycles of detoxification and renewal. **Breath practices**

(Qigong, pranayama) oxygenated the body and cleared stagnation. **Grounding**—barefoot contact with the Earth—reduced inflammation and synced circadian rhythms.

The Vikings? They cold plunged, fermented everything, lived outdoors, prayed to higher forces, and moved with the land. That's longevity in motion. **But the real secret to longevity? Joy and purpose**! No supplement can substitute for a life well-lived. The longest-living people in the world have one thing in common: meaning. The Okinawans call it *ikigai*—a reason to wake up. The Sardinians dance and sing together every day. The Nicoyans tend to their gardens, surrounded by loved ones. Purpose is biological. Joy is medicine. Connection is your birthright. Longevity isn't just in your genes—it's in your daily rhythm.

YOUR VIKING LONGEVITY ACTION PLAN

- ✓ Upgrade your plate: Add wild fish, herbs, fermented foods, mushrooms, and good fats.
- ✓ Supplement smart: Focus on Omega-3s, magnesium, PQQ, glutathione, and tonic herbs.
- ✓ Move and rest: Walk, lift, sweat, and sleep deeply in darkness.
- ✓ Fast occasionally: Give your body space to clean, repair, and renew.
- ✓ Reclaim your rhythm: Sync with the sun, breathe with intention, and ground to the Earth.
- ✓ Live with purpose: Choose joy, mission, and community every day.

You were not born to just grow old—you were born to evolve, expand, and lead the way for those who come after you. As a modern Viking, your power is not just in muscle and willpower, but in wisdom, clarity, and longevity. Let your life be the medicine. Let your health be your rebellion. Let your legacy be one of energy, joy, and unstoppable vitality.

VIKING DIET RECIPES

Eat to detox. Eat to rebuild. Eat to remember.

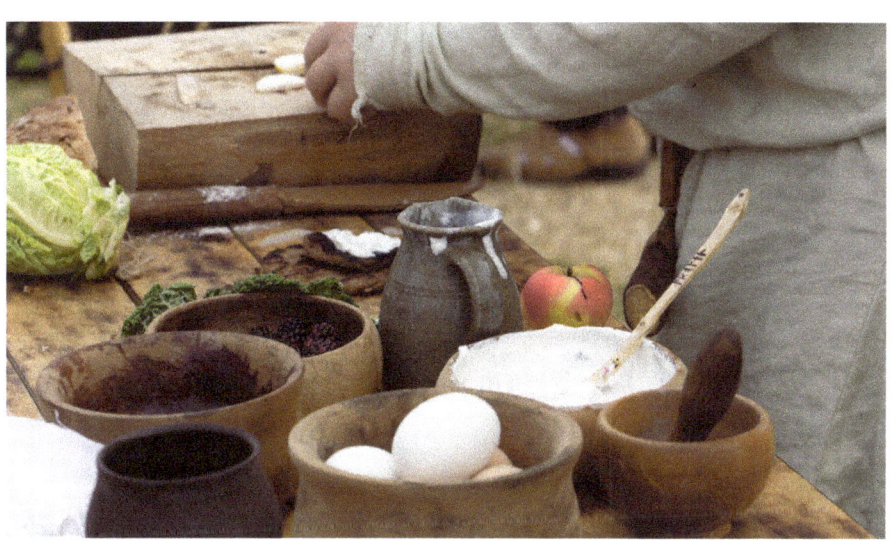

The original Vikings didn't have recipes written down—they cooked by instinct, using what nature gave them in the moment: a freshly caught fish, handpicked mushrooms, a wild herb pulled from the soil. But in today's chaotic world, structure can be your greatest ally. So in this chapter, you'll get a mix of ancient-inspired dishes and modern, nutrient-packed meals to help you live the Viking way—deliciously.

These recipes are designed to be anti-inflammatory, rich in omega-3s and micronutrients, detox-friendly, easy to make, and grounded in nature's cycles. Some are rustic, some are refined, all are functional food that fuels warriors. They are nutrient-dense, earthy, and grounding—with a modern wellness twist.

BREAKFASTS / ENERGY MEALS

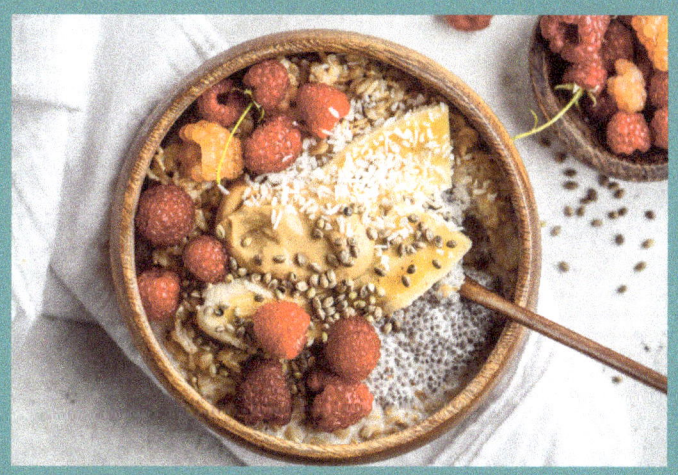

NORDIC CHIA PORRIDGE WITH SEA BUCKTHORN AND PUMPKIN SEEDS

Ingredients:
3 tbsp. chia seeds
1 cup almond or coconut milk
1 tbsp. sea buckthorn puree or lemon zest
1 tbsp. raw honey (optional)

Toppings: pumpkin seeds, hemp seeds, berries

Instructions: Mix chia and milk. Let sit for at least 15 minutes or overnight. Stir in flavorings and top with seeds and berries.

....

PASTURE EGG POWER BOWL WITH PICKLED VEGGIES AND HEMP OIL DRIZZLE

Ingredients:
2–3 pasture-raised eggs
½ avocado, sliced
½ cup cooked lentils or beans
1 handful of arugula
2 tbsp. fermented veggies
1 tsp. hemp oil or flax oil

Instructions: Soft-boil or pan-fry the eggs. Layer ingredients into a bowl, and drizzle oil on top.

....

WILD BERRY AND CHAGA TEA BOWL

A refreshing immune-boosting breakfast bowl

Ingredients:
1 cup cooked fermented oats or barley
½ cup mixed wild berries (fresh or frozen)
½ tsp. cinnamon
½ cup brewed chaga mushroom tea
Drizzle of raw honey

Optional: chia seeds, flax meal

Instructions: Layer the oats and berries, then pour chaga tea over. Drizzle with honey, and sprinkle extras on top.

DETOX AND REPAIR RECIPES FOR MODERN VIKINGS

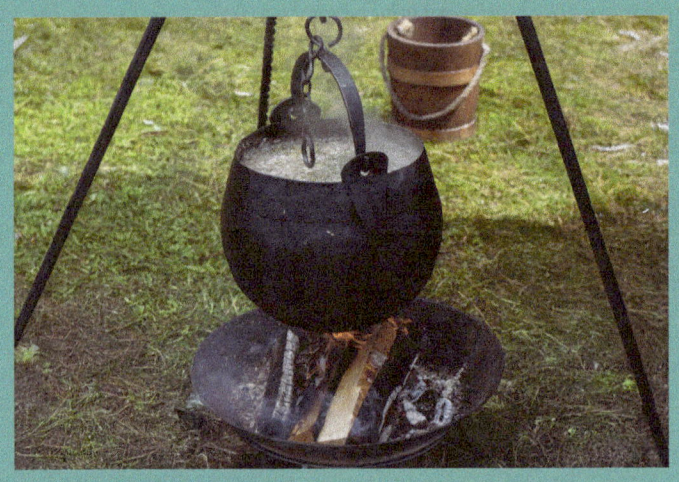

BONE BROTH INFUSION

Ingredients:
2–3 lbs. grass-fed beef or lamb bones (or wild fish heads)
2 tbsp. apple cider vinegar
1 onion
2 carrots
2 celery stalks
Garlic
1 tsp. black peppercorns
Filtered water to cover

Infusion options: Add chaga, ginger, turmeric, lemon peel, or adaptogens like ashwagandha during cooking for a healing upgrade.

Instructions: Simmer in slow cooker 12–24 hrs. (fish: 6 hrs.). Strain and store. Freeze in batches.

· ·

MORNING DETOX ELIXIR

Ingredients:
1 glass warm spring water
Juice of ½ lemon
Pinch of sea salt
Splash of apple cider vinegar

Optional: pinch of cayenne, grated ginger, or activated charcoal (if detoxing)

....

LIVER-LOVING GREEN WARRIOR SMOOTHIE

Ingredients:
1 handful dandelion or arugula
1 handful spinach
½ avocado
½ cup wild blueberries
1 scoop collagen or protein of choice
1 tsp. spirulina or chlorella
Water, coconut water, or unsweetened nut milk

Optional: mint, lime, cilantro for extra liver support
Instructions: Blend and conquer.

....

CHAGA AND REISHI WARRIOR TEA

Ingredients:
1 tbsp. chaga chunks or powder
1 tsp. reishi mushroom powder
1 stick cinnamon

Instructions: Simmer in water 20–40 minutes (or slow-cook overnight). Strain and sip daily as your inner armor.

MITOCHONDRIA BOOSTING POWER SHOT

Great pre-workout or for afternoon energy that doesn't crash

Ingredients:
2 oz. beet juice
1 tsp. shilajit (or a capsule opened into water)
1 capsule PQQ and CoQ10 (optional, if supplementing)
Shot of lemon juice
Tiny pinch of cayenne

LIVER-LOVING GREEN SOUP

Ingredients:
1 bunch dandelion greens or nettle
1 zucchini or celery root, chopped
1 leek or onion, chopped
2 cups vegetable broth
Juice of ½ lemon
1 tbsp. olive oil
Sea salt to taste

Instructions: Sauté onion or leek. Add greens and broth. Simmer 10 minutes, blend until smooth. Stir in lemon juice, olive oil, and serve.

DR. LAURA'S FIRE CIDER

A potent immune tonic, digestive aid, and natural antibiotic—this ancient remedy is one of the strongest plant-based allies for modern Vikings.

Ingredients:
1 cup raw, unfiltered apple cider vinegar
¼ cup grated horseradish root
¼ cup chopped garlic
¼ cup chopped onion
1–2 tbsp. grated fresh ginger
1–2 tbsp. turmeric root (or 1 tsp. powder)
1 lemon, sliced
1–2 tsp. black peppercorns
1 chopped chili pepper (or cayenne to taste)
1–2 tbsp. raw honey (optional, after straining)

Instructions: Combine all ingredients in a large glass jar. Cover with apple cider vinegar (make sure all solids are submerged). Seal with a non-metal lid or use parchment under a metal lid. Let sit in a cool, dark place for 2–4 weeks. Shake daily. Strain, then store in the fridge.

Tips: Take 1–2 tablespoons daily during cold/flu season or at the first sign of illness. Can be used in salad dressings, marinades, or mixed with warm water as a shot.

CHAGA HOT CHOCOLATE

Ingredients:
1 cup brewed chaga tea
1 tbsp. raw cacao powder
½ tsp. cinnamon
1 tsp. coconut oil or ghee
Raw honey or monk fruit, to taste

Instructions: Blend or whisk together and enjoy as a warming adaptogenic tonic.

WARRIOR'S BONE BROTH WITH CHAGA AND BLACK GARLIC

Ingredients:
2 lbs. grass-fed bones or fish heads
1 piece dried chaga (or 1 tbsp. powder)
2 black garlic cloves (or regular garlic)

1 tbsp. apple cider vinegar
2 bay leaves
10 cups water

Instructions: Simmer all ingredients for 12–24 hrs. Strain and store in fridge. Drink warm or use as a soup base.

NETTLE AND ROOT VEGETABLE SOUP

A mineral-rich soup to support the liver, kidneys, and immune system

Ingredients:
2 cups chopped nettle leaves (lightly steamed or blanched if fresh)
1 cup diced carrots
1 cup diced turnips
½ cup leeks or onions
2 garlic cloves, minced
4 cups bone broth or veggie broth
Salt, pepper, and a pinch of dried yarrow or thyme

Instructions: Sauté the onion and garlic, then add the root vegetables and broth. Simmer until tender. Stir in nettles and simmer another 5 minutes. Season and serve.

NETTLE AND LEMON BALM DETOX ELIXIR (KIDNEY AND LIVER SUPPORT)

Ingredients:
1 tsp. dried nettle
1 tsp. lemon balm
½ tsp. fennel seed (optional)
1 slice lemon
1 cup hot water

Instructions: Steep herbs in hot water for 10–15 minutes. Add lemon slice and sip warm.

VIKING CORE MEALS

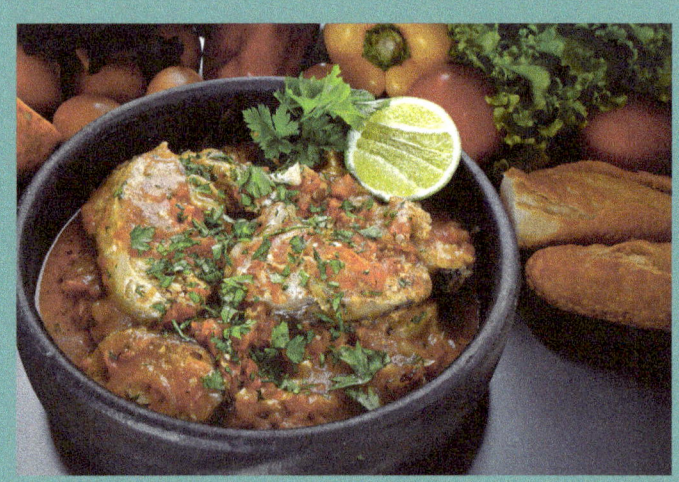

DR. LAURA CAPINA

NORDIC FISHERMAN'S STEW

Ingredients:
1 lb. wild white fish (cod, haddock, or halibut), cubed
1 leek, sliced
2 carrots, chopped
2 potatoes or turnips, cubed
2 cups fish stock or bone broth
1 cup coconut milk (optional, for richness)
2 tbsp. fresh dill, chopped
Sea salt and black pepper to taste
1 tbsp. lemon juice

Instructions: Sauté leeks and carrots in a little olive oil until soft. Add stock and root vegetables; simmer until tender (10–15 minutes). Add fish and simmer gently for another 5–7 minutes. Stir in dill, lemon juice, and coconut milk if using. Serve warm.

....

FERMENTED HERRING WITH BEET SALAD

Ingredients:
2 cooked beets, cubed
½ red onion, finely chopped
2 tbsp. apple cider vinegar
1 tbsp. olive oil
Sea salt and pepper

Store-bought fermented herring (traditional Nordic *surströmming*) or homemade

Optional: chopped dill or horseradish

Instructions: Rinse and slice herring into bite-sized pieces. Layer beet salad on plate, top with fermented herring, and garnish with fresh dill.

· ·

JUNIPER-CRUSTED WILD SALMON

Ingredients:
1 wild-caught salmon fillet
1 tbsp. crushed juniper berries
1 tbsp. olive oil or ghee
1 tsp. sea salt
Fresh dill or parsley for garnish

Instructions: Rub the salmon with oil, salt, and juniper berries. Bake or pan-sear until golden and flaky. Garnish with herbs. Serve with fermented cabbage or root mash.

· ·

DR. LAURA CAPINA

NORDIC ROOT AND BARLEY STEW WITH WILD MUSHROOMS

A grounding, mineral-rich stew inspired by Viking foraging traditions

Ingredients:
1 cup pearl barley (soaked overnight if possible)
1 tbsp. olive oil or ghee
1 onion, chopped
2 garlic cloves, minced
1 carrot, chopped
1 parsnip, chopped
1 cup wild mushrooms (chanterelle, shiitake, or cremini)
1 tsp. sea salt
4 cups vegetable or bone broth
Fresh thyme or dill to finish

Instructions: Sauté onion and garlic in oil until translucent. Add chopped roots and mushrooms. Cook 5–7 minutes. Add soaked barley and broth. Simmer until barley is tender (30–40 minutes). Top with herbs before serving.

· ·

LAMB AND SEAWEED BROTH WITH JUNIPER AND GARLIC

Protein-packed, rich in collagen and iodine—deeply restorative

Ingredients:
1 lb. lamb neck or shank
5–6 cups water
2 garlic cloves
1 small piece kombu or handful dulse
1 tsp. juniper berries
1 bay leaf
Sea salt to taste

Instructions: Simmer lamb in water with garlic and herbs for 2–3 hrs. Add seaweed during the last 30 minutes. Skim fat and serve warm with a drizzle of olive oil.

NORDIC WILD SALMON STEW WITH ROOT VEGGIES AND DILL

Ingredients:
1 lb. wild salmon (skin on)
2 carrots, sliced
1 parsnip or turnip, cubed
1 onion, chopped
2 garlic cloves, minced
1 tbsp. grass-fed butter or olive oil
2 cups bone broth or fish stock
1 tsp. sea salt
1 bunch fresh dill

Optional: splash of coconut milk for creaminess

Instructions: Sauté onions and garlic in butter until soft. Add root veggies and broth. Simmer for 15 minutes. Add salmon and cook gently until just done. Stir in chopped dill before serving.

....

RYE FLATBREAD WITH SMOKED FISH AND NETTLE BUTTER

Flatbread ingredients:
1 cup rye flour
½ tsp. sea salt
½ cup warm water
1 tbsp. olive oil

Instructions: Mix and roll into thin discs, cook on hot dry skillet until both sides are browned.

Nettle butter ingredients:
¼ cup softened grass-fed butter or vegan butter
2 tbsp. steamed and finely chopped nettle leaves
Sea salt to taste

Instructions: Serve flatbread with a smear of nettle butter and slices of smoked fish (trout, mackerel, herring).

....

SEARED ELK (OR GRASS-FED BEEF) WITH JUNIPER BERRY RUB

Ingredients:
1 lb. elk, venison, or grass-fed beef steak
1 tbsp. crushed juniper berries
1 tsp. sea salt
1 tsp. black pepper
1 tbsp. ghee or tallow

Instructions: Rub meat with juniper, salt, and pepper. Sear in hot pan with ghee until medium rare. Rest, slice, and serve with wild greens or fermented veggies.

....

ARCTIC WRAP

A fresh, grounding wrap inspired by northern wild greens and cleansing herbs

Ingredients (makes 2 wraps):
2 sprouted grain wraps or large collard green leaves (blanched)
1 cup shredded red cabbage or sauerkraut
1 cup cooked white beans or lentils
½ cup chopped parsley or dandelion greens
2 tbsp. tahini or nettle hummus
1 small garlic clove, grated
2 tbsp. lemon juice

1 tbsp. olive oil or flax oil
Pinch of sea salt and black pepper

Optional: pickled red onion or thinly sliced cucumber

Instructions: In a bowl, toss the beans/lentils with lemon, oil, garlic, and herbs. Spread tahini on the wrap. Layer with cabbage/sauerkraut and bean mixture. Top with optional vegetables, roll tightly, and slice in half. Serve cold or warm gently on a skillet for a toasty version.

• •

FORAGER'S HERB WRAPS

Leafy wraps using wild greens and herbs

Ingredients:
Large dandelion or kale leaves
½ cup cooked lentils or meat
¼ cup grated carrots
2 tbsp. fermented veggies
1 tsp. crushed wild garlic or dill
Squeeze of lemon

Instructions: Fill each leaf with the mixture and roll them up. Serve cold or lightly warmed. Great for lunch or detox days.

• •

VIKING FLATBREAD
(GRAIN-FREE OR ANCIENT GRAIN OPTION)

Version 1: Ancient Style

Ingredients:
1 cup rye or barley flour
Pinch of salt
½ cup warm water

Instructions: Cook in dry pan like a rustic tortilla.

Version 2: Modern Paleo Style

Ingredients:
1 cup almond flour
2 tbsp. flax meal
1 egg
Pinch of salt

Instructions: Form into flatbreads and bake at 375°F (190°C) for 12 minutes. Top with smoked fish, liver pâté, or honey and bee pollen.

....

DR. LAURA CAPINA

ROASTED ROOT VEGETABLES WITH ANGELICA AND GARLIC

A grounding dish rich in prebiotic fiber and flavor
Ingredients:
1 cup cubed turnips
1 cup carrots
1 small beet
3 garlic cloves
½ tsp. ground Angelica root (or sub with ginger)
Olive oil, sea salt, thyme

Instructions: Toss all ingredients in oil and herbs. Roast at 400°F (200°C) for 30–40 minutes. Serve with sauerkraut or goat cheese.

FERMENTED/GUT HEALING

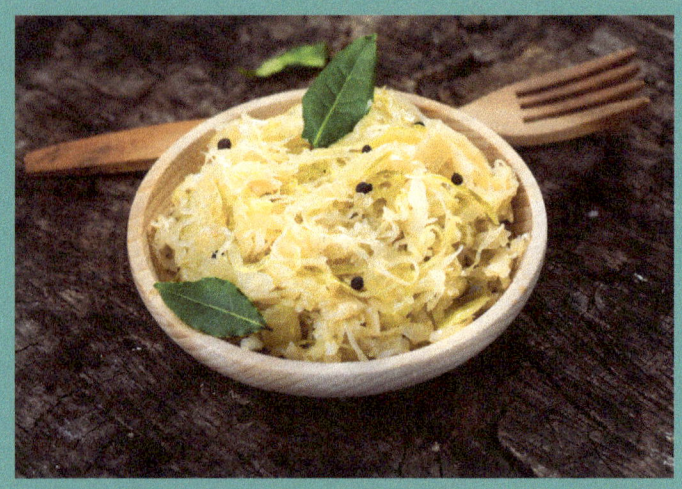

FERMENTED CABBAGE AND ROOT KRAUT (NORDIC SAUERKRAUT)

A daily staple rich in probiotics, enzymes, vitamin C, and digestive fire, this kraut boosts gut health and delivers enzymes critical for digestion.

Ingredients:
1 small head of cabbage, shredded
1 carrot or parsnip, grated
1 tbsp. sea salt (non-iodized)

Optional: caraway seeds, dill, wild garlic, or juniper berries

Instructions: In a large bowl, massage the salt into the cabbage and root veggies until juices release. Pack tightly into a glass jar or crock, pressing down until the brine covers the mixture. Weigh it down (with a clean rock, smaller jar, or fermentation weight). Cover with a cloth or lid (with air escape) and ferment at room temperature for 5–10 days. Taste daily after day four—when tangy and bubbly, it's ready. Store in the fridge for up to 3 months.

....

WILD BERRY AND PURPLE KRAUT FERMENT

Ingredients:
1 small purple cabbage, shredded
½ cup wild blueberries or lingonberries

1 tbsp. sea salt

Instructions: Massage salt into cabbage until juicy. Add berries, mix, and pack into a jar. Cover with brine. Ferment 5–7 days at room temp.

• •

FERMENTED TURNIP "SOUR CHIPS" WITH DILL AND MUSTARD SEED

Ingredients:
1–2 turnips, thinly sliced
1 tbsp. mustard seed
1 clove garlic
1 tbsp. sea salt
2 cups filtered water

Instructions: Dissolve salt in water. Pack turnip slices, garlic, and mustard seed in a jar. Cover with brine. Ferment 3–5 days at room temp.

• •

FERMENTED CABBAGE AND WILD BERRY KRAUT

Add to any meal for a probiotic and polyphenol punch.

Ingredients:
1 small green cabbage, shredded
1 cup wild berries (bilberries or blueberries work great)
1 tbsp. sea salt

Instructions: Massage cabbage and berries with salt until juicy. Pack into a jar, press down tightly, and submerge under its own juice. Cover loosely and ferment at room temperature for 5–7 days.

....

FERMENTED NETTLE TONIC

Ingredients:
1 bunch young nettle leaves
½ cup whey or starter (or probiotic capsule)
1 tsp. sea salt
1 qt. filtered water

Instructions: Pack nettles into a jar. Add salt and starter. Fill with water, leave an inch of headspace. Cover and ferment at room temp for 3–5 days. Strain and refrigerate. Take 2–3 ounces per day.

VIKING MEAD (FERMENTED HONEY WINE)

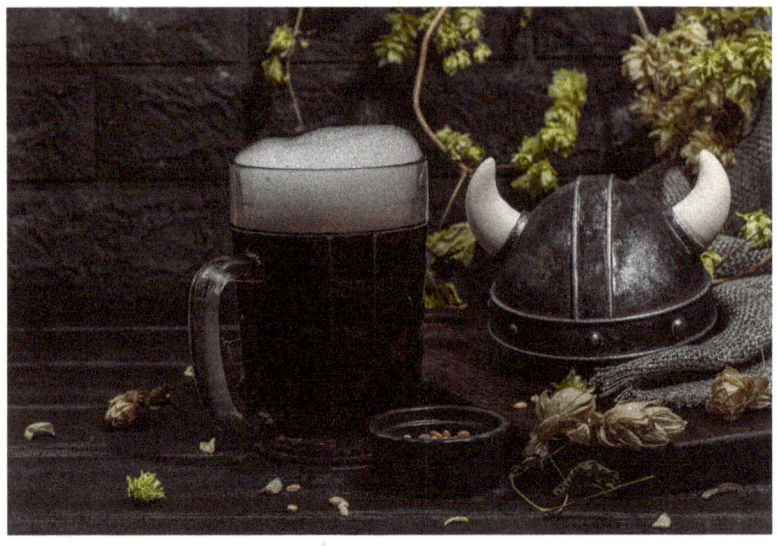

Vikings believed mead was a gift from the gods—reserved for warriors, lovers, and seers. This sacred celebratory and healing drink is rich in enzymes, probiotics, and tradition.

Ingredients:
1 cup raw, unfiltered honey (preferably local)
1 gallon spring water or filtered water
A clean glass fermentation jar or demijohn with airlock

Optional: herbs, like elderflower, yarrow, or mint; wild berries; spices (clove, cinnamon); 1 tsp. wild yeast starter or a pinch of active dry wine/mead yeast
Instructions: Warm about 1 cup of the water and dissolve the honey into it (do not boil). Combine honey-water mixture with the rest of the cold water in the jar. Add

herbs, berries, or spices if using. Stir thoroughly and add yeast if desired. Cover with a breathable cloth (for wild fermentation) or use an airlock if you have one. Let ferment at room temperature (65–75°F/18–24°C) for two to three weeks. Once bubbles slow down and the taste has changed to less sweet and tangier, strain and bottle. Store in the fridge or a cool place. You can let it age for one to three months for more depth.

VIKING-INSPIRED DESSERTS

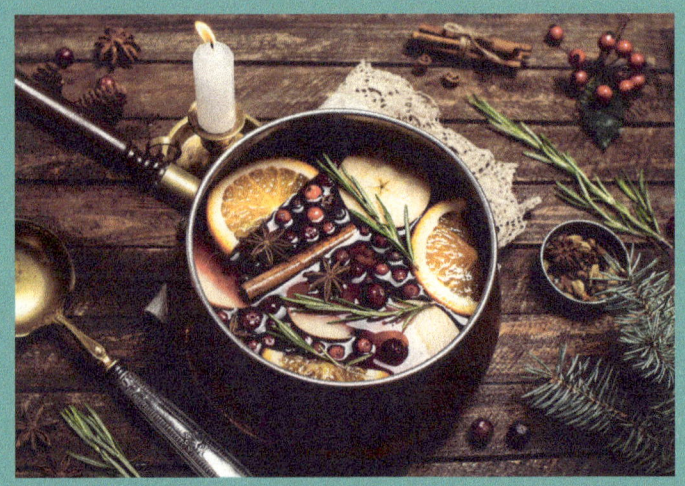

DR. LAURA CAPINA

WARM SPICED APPLE AND BERRY SKILLET

A rustic, skillet-baked treat that feels like a Viking harvest celebration

Ingredients:
2 apples, sliced thin
1 cup mixed berries (fresh or frozen)
1 tbsp. coconut oil or grass-fed butter
1 tsp. cinnamon
¼ tsp. cardamom
1 tsp. lemon juice
1 tbsp. honey or maple syrup (optional)
Pinch of sea salt

Optional: chopped walnuts or hazelnuts

Instructions: In a cast iron skillet, warm the oil/butter over medium heat. Add apples and sauté for 3–5 minutes. Add berries, spices, lemon juice, and a splash of water. Cover and simmer 5 minutes until soft and bubbling. Stir in sweetener if using. Top with chopped nuts. Serve warm as is or with a spoonful of cultured coconut cream or yogurt.

• •

WILD BERRY COMPOTE

Ingredients:
2 cups wild berries (bilberries, lingonberries, blueberries)

1 tbsp. raw honey or birch syrup
1 tsp. lemon zest
1 tsp. chia seeds (optional, for thickening)

Instructions: Simmer berries over low heat for 10 minutes. Stir in lemon zest, chia, and honey after removing from heat. Let cool and store in the fridge.

Tip: This is great over porridge or crispbread.

VIKING CHOCOLATE VITALITY BITES

A rich, energizing, antioxidant treat—perfect after cold plunges or saunas

Ingredients:
1 cup almond flour or ground sunflower seeds
¼ cup raw cacao powder
2 tbsp. tahini or nut butter
1 tbsp. coconut oil
1–2 tbsp. raw honey
½ tsp. cinnamon
¼ tsp. sea salt

Optional: 1 tbsp. ground flax or chia, chopped dried wild berries

Instructions: Mix all ingredients into a thick dough. Roll into small bites or press into a lined pan and chill to firm. Store in fridge or freezer. Eat one to two for a grounding, energizing snack.

....

WILD ROSE AND HONEY BLISS BALLS

A floral, heart-opening dessert that honors the feminine energy of the forest

Ingredients:
1 cup shredded coconut
½ cup almond flour or ground sunflower seeds
2 tbsp. dried wild rose petals (culinary grade)
2 tbsp. raw honey
1 tbsp. coconut oil
1 tsp. vanilla extract
Pinch of sea salt

Optional: 1 tsp. rose water

Instructions: In a food processor, blend all ingredients until a soft dough forms. Roll into small bites and refrigerate until firm. Optional: Roll in crushed rose petals or shredded coconut to finish. Store in the fridge for up to one week.

....

ELDERBERRY MOLASSES BITES

A deep, immune-supportive sweet with Viking apothecary roots

Ingredients:
¾ cup ground walnuts or hemp seeds
2 tbsp. elderberry syrup or concentrate
1 tbsp. blackstrap molasses
1 tbsp. flaxseed meal
1 tsp. cinnamon
¼ tsp. clove

Optional: dried figs or dates for texture

Instructions: Mix all ingredients in a bowl or processor until sticky. Roll into small balls or press into molds. Chill until set. Store in the fridge.

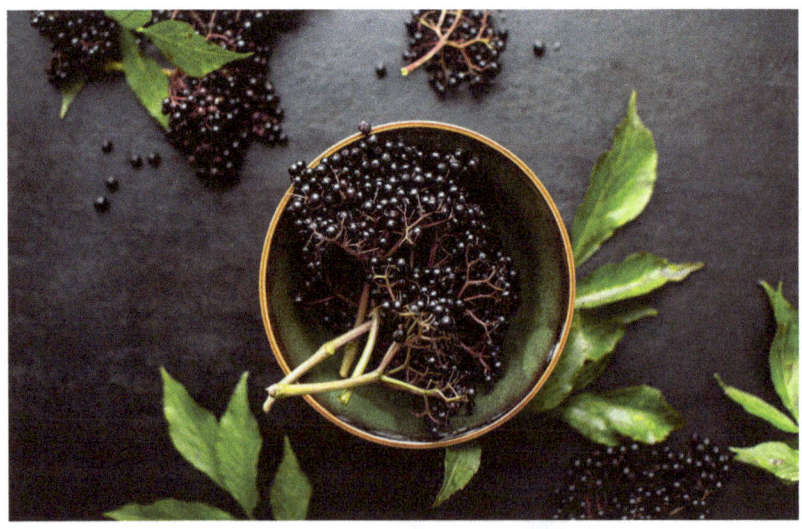

SAMPLE VIKING DAY OF EATING (MODERN VERSION)

Morning:
- ✓ Warm Detox Elixir
- ✓ Viking smoothie or pasture-raised eggs with greens and avocado
- ✓ Herbal tea (chaga, green tea, or pine needle)

Midday:
- ✓ Wild salmon or mackerel salad with fermented veggies, berries, and olive oil
- ✓ Handful of walnuts or Brazil nuts

Afternoon:
- ✓ Bone broth with reishi or medicinal herbs
- ✓ Optional: shilajit or liver capsule for power

Dinner:
- ✓ Grass-fed meat or wild fish
- ✓ Roasted root veggies and sautéed bitter greens
- ✓ Herbal tea or lemon water with minerals

EAT LIKE YOU REMEMBER WHO YOU ARE

These meals are more than fuel. They're rituals. They're the bridge between your ancestors and your highest self. They connect your body to the earth and your spirit to the wild. You don't need a thousand recipes. You need a few powerful ones—made with quality, consciousness, and intention.

PLANT-BASED POWER— THE VIKING DIET FOR VEGANS

*Honor your values. Fuel your strength.
Let the forest feed you.*

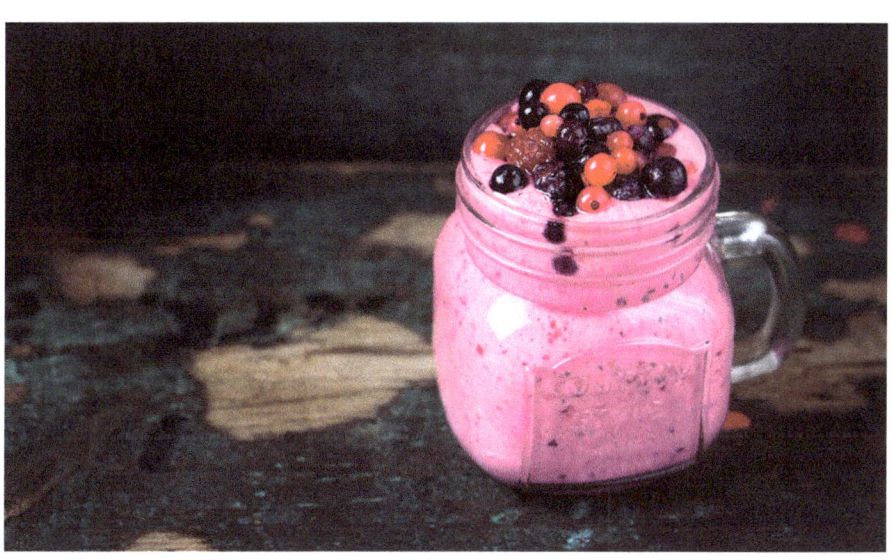

Not all Vikings ate meat every day—and not all modern Vikings need to. While traditional Viking culture was heavily centered around animal foods for survival, the spirit of the *Viking Diet* is about resilience, connection to nature, and nutrient density—not dogma.

In today's world, many people thrive on a plant-based lifestyle when done correctly: with deep intention, variety, and support from functional foods, herbs, and smart supplementation. Though many of the recipes in the previous chapter can be adapted for the vegan Viking, the following recipes are for you if you eat vegan or mostly plant-based, want to honor your body without compromising your ethics, and still want to live strong, wild, detoxed, and vital—like a Viking.

VIKING VEGAN MEAL IDEAS AND RECIPES

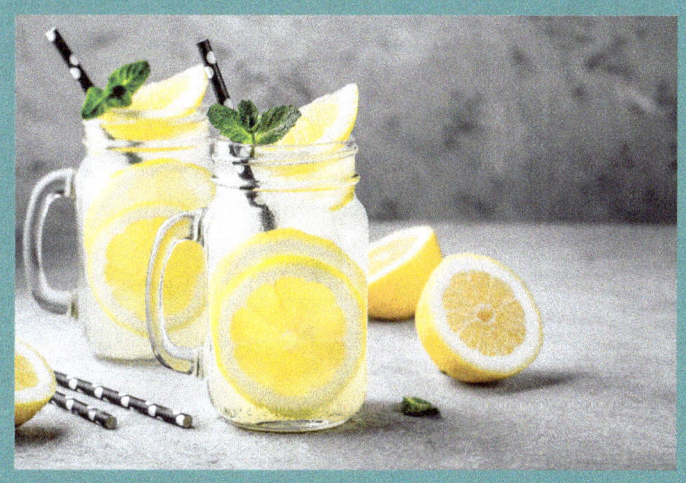

DAILY DETOX ELIXIR

Ingredients:
1 cup warm water
Juice of ½ lemon
Pinch of air-dried sea salt
1 tsp. apple cider vinegar

Optional: 1 capsule of bentonite clay or activated charcoal (empty into water)

Instructions: Drink on an empty stomach in the morning.

．．

CHAGA CHAI WITH COCONUT MILK

Ingredients:
1 cup brewed chaga tea (simmer chaga chunks or powder for 30–60 minutes)
1 cup unsweetened coconut milk
½ tsp. cinnamon
¼ tsp. cardamom
¼ tsp. ginger powder
Pinch of black pepper
1–2 tsp. maple syrup or coconut sugar

Optional: dash of vanilla or star anise

Instructions: Brew chaga tea separately (strong is best). Warm coconut milk in a pot with spices. Whisk together with chaga tea and sweetener. Strain if needed and froth for a creamy finish.

....

GOLDEN MILK (VEGAN TURMERIC LATTE)

A soothing, anti-inflammatory bedtime tonic with deep ancestral roots

Ingredients (1 serving):
1 cup coconut milk or almond milk
½ tsp. turmeric powder
¼ tsp. cinnamon
Pinch of black pepper (boosts curcumin absorption)
¼ tsp. ginger powder or 1 tsp. fresh grated
1 tsp. coconut oil (optional for richness)
1 tsp. maple syrup or raw honey (if not strictly vegan)

Optional: pinch of cardamom or dash of vanilla; add a dash of ashwagandha powder or reishi extract for stress relief and nervous system nourishment.

Instructions: In a small saucepan, whisk all ingredients together. Heat gently (do not boil), whisking until warm and slightly frothy. Pour into a mug and sip slowly, ideally before bed or during a wind-down ritual.

WILD BERRY NETTLE PORRIDGE

A mineral-rich, earthy breakfast inspired by Nordic forest mornings

Ingredients:
½ cup gluten-free oats or buckwheat groats
1 tbsp. ground flax or chia seeds
1 tsp. dried nettle powder or 2 tbsp. fresh steamed nettle
1 cup plant milk (coconut, hemp, or almond)
½ cup wild berries (lingonberries, bilberries, blueberries)
1 tsp. cinnamon
1–2 tsp. birch syrup or maple syrup
Pinch of sea salt

Instructions: In a pot, combine oats, plant milk, nettle, flax, salt, and cinnamon. Simmer 5–8 minutes. Stir in berries and sweetener, cook another 2 minutes. Serve topped with extra berries, seeds, or a drizzle of nut butter.

· ·

VIKING FOREST SMOOTHIE BOWL

A detox-friendly breakfast with adaptogens, greens, and healthy fats

Ingredients:
1 frozen banana
1 tsp. spirulina or chlorella

1 tsp. reishi or chaga mushroom powder
1 tbsp. hemp seeds or flax oil
1 scoop plant-based protein (optional)
½ cup frozen zucchini or cauliflower (optional, for creaminess)
¾ cup coconut or almond milk
Juice of ½ lemon

Toppings: wild berries, pumpkin seeds, coconut flakes, nettle powder sprinkle, or granola

Instructions: Blend all base ingredients until smooth and thick. Pour into a bowl and decorate with toppings. Eat slowly, with intention—it's as much a ritual as a meal.

• •

WARM ROOT BOWL WITH FERMENTED CABBAGE AND HEMP SEEDS

Ingredients:
1 sweet potato, roasted
1 carrot and beet, shredded
½ cup sauerkraut or kimchi
2 tbsp. hemp seeds
Handful of arugula

Dressing: tahini, lemon, garlic, sea salt

Instructions: Roast sweet potato until tender. Assemble bowl with all ingredients. Drizzle with dressing and top with seeds.

....

NETTLE AND LENTIL SOUP WITH GARLIC AND MISO

Nourishing, grounding, and immune-boosting

Ingredients:
1 cup cooked green or black lentils
2 cups fresh nettle or spinach
1 tbsp. miso paste
3 garlic cloves
1 tbsp. olive oil
1 tsp. cumin
Water or veggie broth
Instructions: Sauté garlic in olive oil. Add broth, lentils, greens, spices—simmer 10–15 minutes. Stir in miso at the end (don't boil miso).

....

MINERAL BROTH WITH NETTLE AND SHIITAKE

Ingredients:
1 bunch nettle (or kale/dandelion)
½ cup dried shiitake mushrooms

1 onion and garlic
1 carrot and celery stalk
1 piece kombu (optional)
2 tsp. apple cider vinegar
Sea salt and herbs to taste

Instructions: Simmer all ingredients for 1–2 hrs. Strain and sip as a mineral-rich tonic.

• •

DETOX WARRIOR SMOOTHIE BOWL

Ingredients:
½ banana
½ avocado
1 handful wild blueberries
1 tsp. spirulina or chlorella
1 scoop plant protein
1 tbsp. chia or flax
Almond or coconut milk

Instructions: Assemble, then top with pumpkin seeds, shredded coconut, and/or cacao nibs.

• •

VIKING SEAWEED SALAD WITH LEMON–GINGER DRESSING

Mineral-rich, alkalizing, great for thyroid and detox

Ingredients:
½ cup soaked wakame or dulse
Sliced cucumber and radish
Handful of shredded carrots
Dressing: sesame oil, lemon, grated ginger, tamari

....

MUSHROOM AND WALNUT "MEAT" WRAPS

Protein-packed, satisfying, and deliciously primal

Ingredients:
1 cup mushrooms, finely chopped
½ cup walnuts, pulsed in food processor
1 tsp. cumin, garlic, and sea salt
Lettuce leaves or grain-free wrap

Instructions: Sauté mushrooms in olive oil with seasoning. Mix in walnuts and serve in wraps with avocado, herbs, or kraut.

....

DR. LAURA CAPINA

SMOKY BEETROOT AND WALNUT TARTARE

A grounding vegan dish that mimics liver's depth with a clean, earthy twist

Ingredients:
2 small roasted beets, grated
½ cup walnuts, finely chopped
1 tbsp. olive oil
1 tsp. smoked paprika
½ tsp. tamari or coconut aminos
1 tbsp. lemon juice
Pinch of sea salt and black pepper

Instructions: Mix all ingredients and let sit 10 minutes before serving. Serve on rye toast, flatbread, or crisp greens.

···

STUFFED SWEET POTATO

A grounding, nutrient-rich dinner that feels indulgent—but deeply detoxifying

Ingredients (serves 1–2):
1 large sweet potato, baked
1 cup sautéed kale or chard (with garlic and olive oil)
½ cup cooked lentils or chickpeas
1 tbsp. coconut yogurt or tahini

Optional: turmeric, cumin, black sesame seeds, chopped fresh herbs, sea salt, lemon

Instructions: Bake sweet potato at 400°F (200°C) for 45–60 minutes or until soft. While baking, sauté greens and warm lentils with your favorite spices. Slice sweet potato open, mash the inside slightly with a fork. Pile on the greens and lentils, drizzle with yogurt or tahini. Garnish with sesame seeds and herbs. Add a pinch of sea salt and squeeze of lemon for extra flavor and digestion.

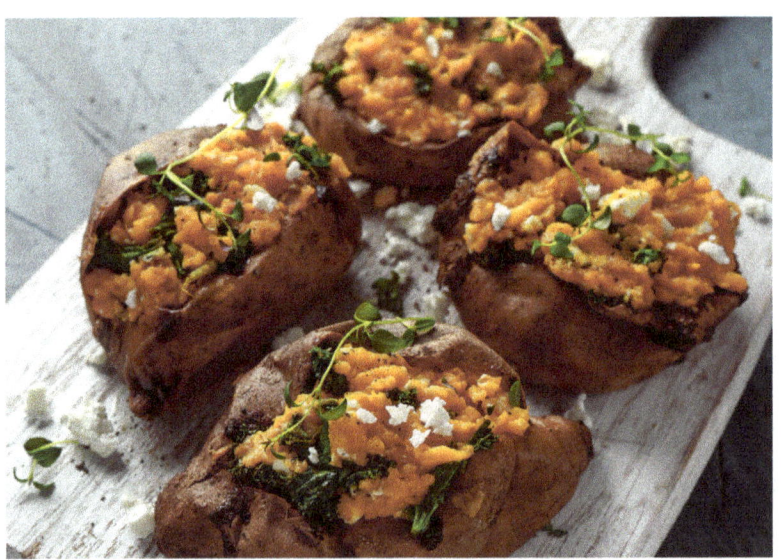

DR. LAURA CAPINA

CHICKPEA AND DANDELION PATTIES WITH FERMENTED VEG SLAW

Ingredients (Patties):
1 can chickpeas, rinsed
1 cup dandelion greens, chopped
2 garlic cloves
2 tbsp. ground flax
½ tsp. cumin
½ tsp. sea salt
½ tsp. black pepper
1 tbsp. olive oil for frying

Instructions: Pulse all ingredients (except oil) in a food processor. Form into patties and pan-fry until golden on both sides. For the slaw: Shred cabbage, carrot, and 2 tbsp. sauerkraut. Toss with lemon and flax oil.

....

WILD BERRY AND BEET FERMENT

Ingredients:
1 cup shredded raw beet
½ cup wild berries
1 tsp. grated ginger
1 tsp. sea salt
Starter or brine from sauerkraut

Instructions: Pack into glass jar. Add salt and starter. Cover with cabbage leaf or weight. Ferment five to seven days. Refrigerate and eat 1 tbsp./day.

NORDIC SEED CRISPBREAD

Ingredients:
½ cup sunflower seeds
¼ cup flaxseeds
¼ cup sesame seeds
¼ cup pumpkin seeds
¼ cup chia seeds
1 cup water
½ tsp. sea salt

Instructions: Soak seeds for 1 hr. Spread thin on parchment, then bake 300°F (150°C) for 30–40 minutes until crisp. Break into pieces. Store dry.

VEGAN DESSERTS

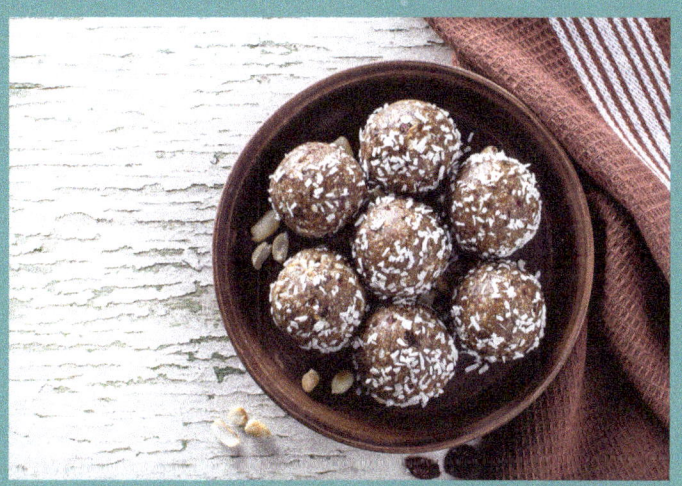

RAW CACAO AND SEA SALT ENERGY BITES

Rich in magnesium and antioxidants—perfect Viking fuel

Ingredients:
1 cup dates, pitted
½ cup raw almonds or walnuts
¼ cup raw cacao powder
1 tbsp. flax or chia seeds
Pinch of sea salt
1 tsp. vanilla
1 tbsp. coconut oil (optional)

Instructions: Blend all ingredients in food processor until sticky. Roll into balls. Dust with cacao or coconut. Chill in fridge. Keeps 1–2 weeks.

....

WILD BERRY AND COCONUT CHIA PARFAIT

Inspired by Nordic berries and creamy layered textures

Ingredients:
1 cup full-fat coconut milk
2 tbsp. chia seeds
1 tbsp. maple syrup or birch syrup
½ tsp. vanilla
½ cup mashed wild berries (bilberries, lingonberries, blueberries)

Instructions: Mix coconut milk, chia, syrup, and vanilla. Let sit 20 minutes or overnight. Layer chia pudding with mashed berries in a glass. Garnish with dried berries or shaved coconut.

NETTLE AND HAZELNUT BLISS BARS

A sweet way to sneak in mineral-rich greens

Ingredients:
½ cup ground hazelnuts
½ cup oats
2 tbsp. dried nettle powder or matcha
¼ cup almond butter
2 tbsp. maple syrup
Pinch of sea salt

Optional: melted vegan chocolate to drizzle

Instructions: Mix all ingredients until sticky. Press into pan, chill until firm. Slice into bars and drizzle with chocolate if desired.

SPICED APPLE AND CARAWAY SKILLET CRISP

Old world flavor with modern nourishment

Ingredients:
2 apples, sliced
1 tsp. lemon juice
½ tsp. cinnamon
¼ tsp. cardamom
1 tbsp. maple syrup

Topping:
½ cup oats
2 tbsp. almond flour
2 tbsp. coconut oil or vegan butter
1 tsp. caraway seeds
1 tbsp. coconut sugar

Instructions: Toss apples with lemon, spices, and maple. Add to skillet. Combine topping and sprinkle over apples. Bake at 350°F (175°C) for 25–30 minutes until golden and soft. Serve warm with coconut yogurt or coconut milk drizzle.

TIPS FOR VEGAN VIKINGS

Supplement wisely: B12, DHA (from algae), zinc, iron, and vitamin D are often needed. Prioritize fermented and sprouted foods to ease digestion and increase absorption. Soak legumes, grains, and seeds to reduce anti-nutrients. Use adaptogens and medicinal mushrooms for hormonal and nervous system support.

Remember: Viking is a vibe, not a rulebook. Whether you eat plants or animals or both, the real Viking diet is about choosing foods that come from the earth, avoiding what is processed, fake, and toxic, and eating with purpose, strength, and reverence. You can be a vegan Viking—wild, detoxed, rooted, and unstoppable.

WHAT SHOULD I EAT? PERSONALIZED NUTRITION

There's no one-size-fits-all—only one-size-fits-YOU.

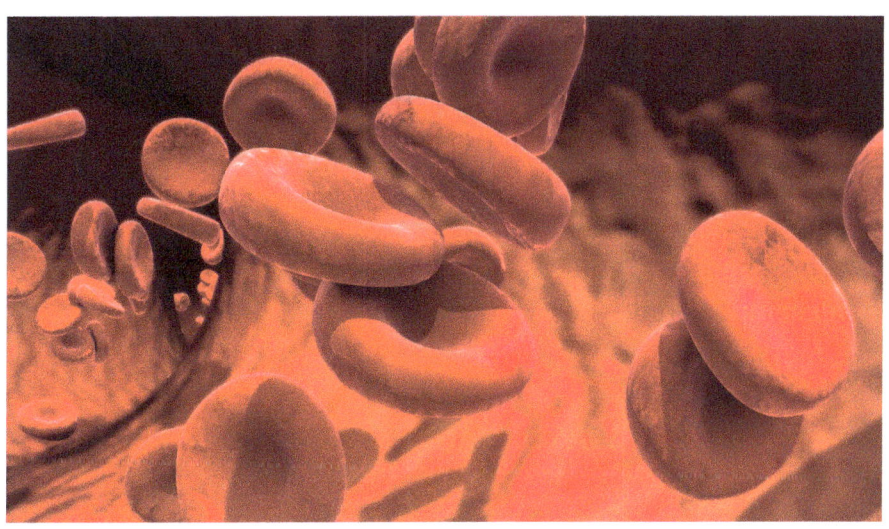

"Just tell me what to eat" is one of the most common statements I get from patients. And while I understand the desire for a simple plan, the truth is, you are not a formula. You are a constellation of ancestry, metabolism, climate, lifestyle, age, and soul design. But here's the good news: You can always upgrade from where you are.

Whether you're eating fast food or already organic, there's always a next level.

START WHERE YOU ARE: FOOD QUALITY UPGRADES

It's not about being perfect. It's about gradual elevation.

- Bread? Go from white → whole wheat → organic sourdough → sprouted flourless grain
- Meat? Start from conventional → cage free → pasture-raised → 100 percent grass-fed
- Oil? Ditch canola → use cold-pressed olive, avocado, flax, or coconut
- Water? Trade tap → filtered → spring → mineral-rich, structured water

This approach removes the shame and allows transformation to feel empowering—not overwhelming.

CLIMATE, SEASON, AND LOCATION MATTER

What you need depends on where you live. In **cold northern climates**, favor warming, grounding foods: soups, stews, meats, root vegetables, and herbs like rosemary and ginger. In **hot, humid environments**: Choose cooling, hydrating foods, like cucumbers, watermelon, berries, mint, and leafy greens. Winter requires more fat and warmth. Summer thrives on light, water-rich foods. This is how humans have always eaten—with the Earth, not against it.

LIFESTYLE AND LABOR

What you do determines what you need. **Mental labor** (computers, students, executives) needs healthy fats like omega-3s, avocados, walnuts, olives, DHA-rich algae oil—fuel for the brain, nerves, and EMF protection. **Physical labor** (construction, athletes, manual workers) needs more protein, electrolytes, and complex carbs to repair tissue and maintain stamina. **Stressful lifestyles** need adaptogens, minerals, and extra magnesium.

FEMALE LIFE STAGE NUTRITION

Pregnancy and nursing: You're not eating for two—you're building one. Key nutrients include omega-3s (especially DHA), B vitamins, folate, magnesium, iron, choline, and collagen (for tissue repair). Bone broth, liver (or plant-based B12), wild salmon, greens, and superfood smoothies are excellent.

MENOPAUSE: HORMONES ARE CHANGING—BUT THAT'S NOT A DISEASE, IT'S A TRANSFORMATION.

Prioritize omega-3s and vitamin E (for mood, skin, and heart); flax, maca, sesame (phytohormone balancing); protein to prevent sarcopenia; magnesium, D3/K2, and adaptogens for bone, sleep, and stress; and bitter greens and fiber for estrogen detox.

BLOOD TYPE AND ANCESTRAL BLUEPRINT

There's science suggesting that blood type affects digestive enzymes and immune reactions to food. **Type O** thrives on higher-protein, ancestral diets with meat and fish. **Type A** does well with more vegetarian foods, grains, and legumes. **Type B** is a mix and often tolerates dairy better. **Type AB** is flexible but needs digestive support. These are not rigid rules, but a lens to consider, especially for long-standing digestive or immune challenges.

AYURVEDIC DOSHAS: ANCIENT BIO-INDIVIDUALITY

Ayurveda teaches that we're each made of different elemental forces:

- Vata (air/ether): cold, dry, light → needs grounding, warm, moist food (soups, oils, stews)
- Pitta (fire/water): hot, intense → needs cooling, calming food (greens, cucumbers, coconut, herbs)
- Kapha (earth/water): heavy, slow → needs light, spicy, bitter food (leafy greens, chili, ginger, turmeric)

Tuning into your dominant dosha can clarify why some foods energize you and others make you sluggish.

AGE AND NUTRITIONAL NEEDS

Children and teens need protein, omega-3s, and minerals (especially calcium, zinc, magnesium) for growth and brain development. **Young adults** need detox support, hormone balance, adaptogens, and B vitamins. Those in **midlife** need anti-inflammatory support, blood sugar stability, and cognitive nutrients, whereas **elders** require mitochondrial support (CoQ10, PQQ, NAD precursors), omega-3s, and nutrient absorption support (enzymes, bitters, minerals).

UNIVERSAL TEMPLATES: MEAL PLANS THAT WORK FOR MOST

Whether you eat three meals a day or practice intermittent fasting, what matters most is what you eat and how you feel. The older we get, the less we may need—but the higher the quality must be.

Some people thrive on three structured meals. Others do best with one or two nutrient-dense meals per day and an herbal tonic in between. This section provides flexible, functional templates that can be adapted to all rhythms and seasons of life.

Breakfast Options (or break fast around 10–11 a.m. if practicing intermittent fasting)

Wild Berry Nettle Porridge

» Made with soaked oats or buckwheat, chia seeds, and simmered in coconut milk or water
» Stir in dried nettle powder, flaxseeds, cinnamon, and top with wild berries and walnuts.
» Rich in minerals, fiber, and antioxidants—great for grounding and focus

Green Smoothie Bowl

- » Blend spinach, frozen zucchini or banana, wild blueberries, flax oil, and plant-based protein.
- » Add spirulina or chlorella for detox support.
- » Top with pumpkin seeds, coconut flakes, and nettle powder for extra nourishment.

Warm Broth Breakfast (for light eaters or intermittent fasters)

- » Sip bone broth or mineral broth with a drizzle of flax or MCT oil.
- » Add kelp flakes, reishi powder, or a soft-boiled egg (if not fully plant-based).
- » Perfect for deep gut healing, hydration, and morning calm

Savory Rye Toast with Nettle Butter

- » Toast sprouted rye or seed bread.
- » Spread with nettle herb butter or hummus, and top with radish or sauerkraut.
- » Add avocado or smoked mushrooms for extra depth.
- » Intermittent Fasting Tip: If you're skipping breakfast, begin the day with lemon water, herbal tea, minerals, or a gentle tonic like chaga chai or the Daily Detox Elixir.

Lunch Ideas (your main meal if you're doing 16:8 fasting or have higher activity midday)

Modern Viking Bowl

» Base: quinoa, wild rice, or steamed root vegetables
» Add sautéed greens (dandelion, arugula), fermented veggies, wild salmon or lentils.
» Drizzle with flax oil, lemon, and fresh herbs.

Soup and Crispbread Combo

» Liver-Loving Green Soup with kale, zucchini, nettle, and lemon
» Nordic Seed Crispbread with hummus, avocado, and microgreens
» Add a side of fermented beets or carrot sticks.

Arctic Wrap

» Use sprouted grain or lettuce leaf as the wrap.
» Fill with shredded cabbage, white beans, parsley, tahini, garlic, and pickled onions.
» Balances gut health, protein, and bitter greens

Wild Greens and Detox Plate

» ½ greens (steamed or raw): arugula, nettle, or dandelion
» ¼ clean protein: lentils, tempeh, wild fish, or hemp seeds
» ¼ fat-rich side: avocado, olives, seed mix
» Optional: roasted carrots, turmeric potatoes, sauerkraut

Brainworkers: Add walnuts, algae oil, or reishi powder for mental clarity. Labor-intensive days: Add extra protein and starchy roots like sweet potatoes.

Dinner Options (light and easy to digest—ideal around sunset or 3–4 hrs. before bed)

Nordic Vegetable Stew

- Simmer carrots, celery, turnips, and mushrooms in mineral broth.
- Add garlic, bay leaf, seaweed, and a spoonful of miso or tahini.
- Gentle, warming, and restorative

Stuffed Sweet Potato

- Roast whole sweet potato and fill with sautéed kale, lentils, garlic, and coconut yogurt drizzle.
- Optional: chopped herbs and pomegranate for brightness

Herbal Grain Bowl

- Base of buckwheat or millet
- Top with steamed broccoli, wild mushrooms, and fermented cabbage.
- Sprinkle with pumpkin seeds, turmeric, and a squeeze of lemon.

Evening Elixir Meal (for light eaters or elders)

- » Sip on Chaga Hot Chocolate or Golden Milk.
- » Pair with a small bowl of mashed avocado on a seed cracker or a warm apple and walnut bake.
- » Ideal for those who eat once or twice daily and prioritize digestion and sleep

Tip: As we age, it's wise to eat less at night to support sleep, detox, and hormone repair. A light, warm meal supports the liver and circadian rhythm.

YOUR BODY IS THE GUIDE

There is no single perfect diet. But there is one perfect principle: Listen, respond, evolve. Upgrade your food quality. Adapt based on your body, season, and lifestyle. And when in doubt—choose what's alive, whole, and closest to nature.

Your body has wisdom. Your ancestors left clues. This book is your map—but the path is yours.

THE PATH FORWARD—BECOME THE VIKING YOUR ANCESTORS KNEW YOU COULD BE

"You must be the change you wish to see in the world." –Gandhi

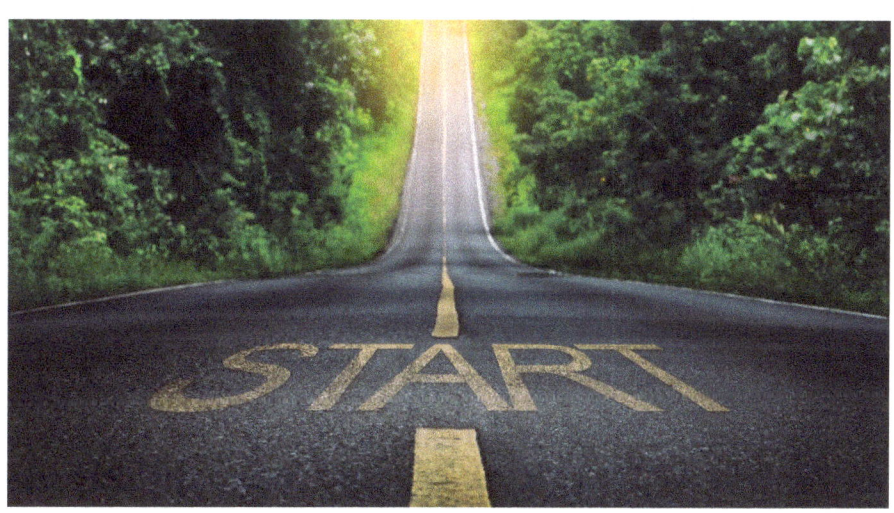

You were never meant to be weak. You were never meant to be sick, inflamed, foggy, anxious, or disconnected.

You were meant to be strong. You were designed to be clear, vital, grounded, and alive. You carry the DNA of warriors, healers, explorers, and survivors.

The modern world tries to tame that fire—through toxic food, synthetic living, overstimulation, distraction, and disconnection. But deep down, you've always known: This isn't how we're supposed to live. That's why you're here.

The Modern Viking Diet is not just about what to eat. It's about how to live with honor, vitality, and sovereignty in a world that's lost its way. It's about reclaiming your connection to the earth beneath your feet, the food that fuels your body, the breath that calms your mind, the rituals that ground your spirit, and the wild strength that has always lived within you.

Whether you eat meat or plants, whether you live in the city or forest, whether you're just starting or already deep on your path—this way of life is available to you. You now have the blueprint, but this book isn't a finish line—it's a beginning. A doorway back to yourself.

YOU ARE THE ONE YOU'VE BEEN WAITING FOR

By now, you've uncovered the hidden truths about how your body actually works … how toxins accumulate and how to release them … how to nourish yourself with food that heals, not harms … and how to return to your natural state of strength, clarity, and resilience. You now have the tools, the maps, the rituals, the clarity—but the most powerful tool of all is you.

This book is not a set of rules. It's a mirror and a compass. It reflects who you are capable of becoming—and it points you back to the path you were always meant to walk. And the path is this:

You are responsible for your health. Not your doctor. Not the food industry. Not your genetics. You. That's not a burden. That's your greatest power.

Responsibility is not about blame. It's about ownership. The moment you take full responsibility for your well-being, your life begins to transform. And here's the truth: You don't need to do everything at once. In fact, the greatest transformations begin with one powerful step.

When you tell yourself, "I choose this"—your brain shifts. When you say, "This is who I am now"—your identity upgrades. Change doesn't come from force. It comes from alignment. And alignment begins the moment you say, "This is the life I will live. This is the body I choose to have. This is the legacy I will leave."

CONSISTENCY OVER PERFECTION

I've seen it time and time again in my practice—just one or two consistent upgrades can change everything.

- ✓ Swap one toxic product for a clean one.
- ✓ Drink lemon water before your coffee.
- ✓ Add omega-3s daily.
- ✓ Take five deep breaths before a meal.
- ✓ Go for a walk instead of scrolling.
- ✓ Say "no" to what drains you and "yes" to what lights you up.

The key is consistency. The magic is momentum. And the power? That's already inside you.

DO IT FOR YOU. DO IT FOR THEM. DO IT FOR THE PLANET.

You're not just healing for yourself. You're becoming stronger so your children, your community, and even your future grandchildren can live in a healthier world.

We need leaders who walk with clarity. We need parents who model vitality. We need elders who radiate peace, not pain.

You doing this work—right now—matters more than you know. This is how we change the world. Not through politics, not through fear, but through energy, action and alignment.

CLOSING ACTIVATION

Let this next part land deep in your subconscious. Take a moment and breathe, then imagine yourself six months from now—standing taller, thinking clearer, radiating peace. Your energy is strong. Your body is light. Your heart is open. You've become the version of yourself you always knew you could be. You are the storm and the stillness. You are the healer and the healed. You are the Viking of your own destiny. Now close your eyes and really feel this in your every cell—and start living like it.

Take what you've learned—and live it. Make your life your medicine. Make your days your rituals. Walk through the world like someone whose ancestors are watching and cheering you on. Because they are. Become the Viking your ancestors knew you could be—and may your strength awaken others.

REFLECTIONS

Your Viking journey begins here. Grab a pen or pencil, and take a moment to anchor what you've learned.

What are one to three changes I will start this week?

_____

_____

_____

What am I most excited to improve, and why?

_____

_____

_____

What core principle resonates with me the most, and why?

_____

_____

_____

What does "modern Viking strength" mean to me?

_____

_____

_____

What is my long-term vision for my body, mind, and spirit?

_____

_____

_____

My Top Three Next Steps

1. _____

2. _____

3. _____

My declaration: I commit to reclaiming my health, my strength, and my joy. I am no longer waiting. I am the one I've been waiting for.

METHODOLOGY

This book is not a summary of other books. It's a living synthesis—born from two decades of hands-on clinical practice, ancient wisdom, modern science, and relentless curiosity.

Every page you've read is grounded in something far more powerful than theory: real-world results. I've seen thousands of patients—every age, every condition, every stage of healing—and guided them back to balance using the exact principles shared in these chapters.

My approach is not tied to any single school of thought. Instead, it's a deep integration of the most effective healing systems across time and culture:

- A master's and doctorate in Traditional Chinese Medicine with formal study in China under renowned traditional doctors
- Advanced certifications in Quantum Reflex Analysis (QRA) and Applied Kinesiology-based nutritional testing—personally trained by the late Dr. Bob Marshall, whose methods remain foundational in my diagnostic approach
- Deep immersion in the world's most impactful dietary models, from Mediterranean and South Beach to the Zone, Vegan, and Carnivore—not just reading about them, but critically evaluating what works, what heals, and what harms based on outcomes and lab data

- A childhood shaped by Latvian folk wisdom, wild herbs, forest medicine, and deeply rooted traditions around food, health, and seasonal rhythms
- Continuous exploration of plant medicines from Chinese, Ayurvedic, European, and Amazonian traditions, understanding how different ecosystems provide exactly what the body needs when used with respect and intention
- Attendance at top global events, such as the Biohacking Conference, David Wolfe's Longevity Conference, and training in human potential with Tony Robbins and The Landmark Forum
- And perhaps most importantly, the lessons that no school can teach—the patterns I've witnessed firsthand in clinic; the stories of recovery; the bodies that spoke louder than textbooks; the results that came not from dogma—but from listening, testing, and refining

In building this book, I've also cross-referenced current scientific literature, clinical trials, and health journals—particularly in areas such as detoxification, omega-3 fatty acids, mitochondrial health, hormone regulation, herbal pharmacology, and neuroinflammation. Yes, PubMed was part of my research—but so was the forest, so were my patients, so was my intuition.

The Modern Viking Diet is not a copy of what has been done. It is a fusion of what actually works—rooted in tradition, backed by science, and guided by real healing. And now—it's yours.

ABOUT DR. LAURA

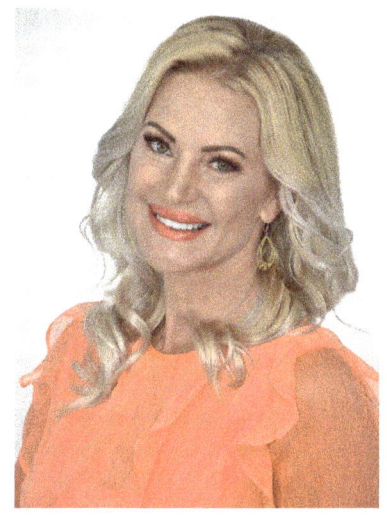

Dr. Laura Capina is a doctor of Chinese Medicine, licensed acupuncturist, herbalist, clinical nutritionist, and wellness educator dedicated to helping people reclaim their health through nature's timeless wisdom.

Born and raised in Latvia, Dr. Laura grew up connected to the Earth—eating wild forest berries, fishing with her uncles, foraging for mushrooms, and drinking birch sap every spring to renew the body after long winters. Her upbringing instilled in her a deep respect for ancestral foods, herbal remedies, and living in rhythm with the seasons.

After moving to the United States in her early twenties, she was shocked by the amount of chronic disease, allergies, and auto-immune conditions she witnessed. This launched her life's mission: to understand why modern people are so sick and learn how to reverse it naturally.

She earned her master's degree and PhD in Chinese Medicine, studying with renowned teachers in China, and has spent nearly two decades treating thousands of patients in clinical practice. She is also a certified quantum reflex analysis (QRA) practitioner under the mentorship of Dr. Bob Marshall, who has taught her no matter what disease label someone carries, the body has only one true foundation—the blueprint created by God.

Dr. Laura combines Eastern medicine, modern nutrition, detoxification science, biohacking insights, and spiritual wisdom to create practical protocols that work. She believes true health is not about extremes or fear—it's about aligning with the laws of nature, strengthening your inner terrain, and living with purpose, resilience, and joy.

Through her writing, teaching, and clinical work, she hopes to awaken the Viking within each of us and encourage us to stand strong, live boldly, and leave a legacy of radiant health for the generations to come.

www.ingramcontent.com/pod-product-compliance
Lightning Source LLC
Chambersburg PA
CBHW060455030426
42337CB00015B/1594